P9-BTO-915

Beginning
Life

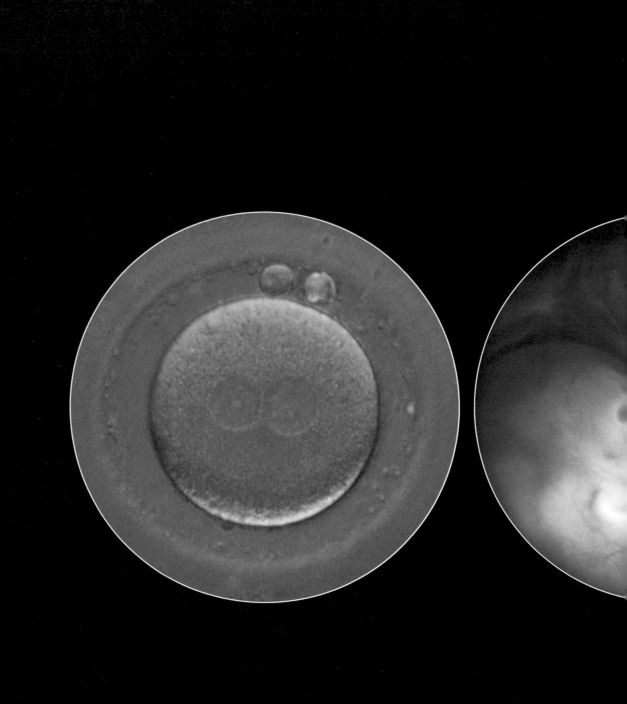

Beginning
Life

Geraldine Lux Flanagan

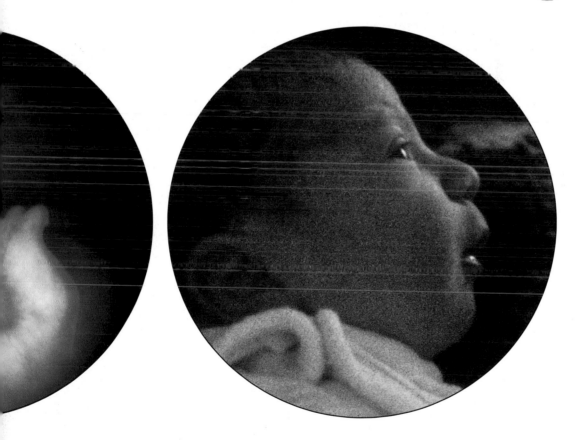

A DK PUBLISHING BOOK

The original concept for this book is the author's
Designer Peter Luff
Editor Gwen Edmonds
US Editor Constance M. Robinson

First American Edition, 1996
2 4 6 8 10 9 7 5 3 1

Published in the United States by
DK Publishing, Inc.
95 Madison Avenue
New York, New York 10016
http://www.dk.com

Library of Congress Cataloging-in-Publication Data

Flanagan, Geraldine Lux.
        Beginning life/by Geraldine Lux Flanagan. –
1st American ed.
                    p. cm.
            Includes index.
            ISBN 0-7894-0609-8
            1. Embryology. Human-Popular works.
                I. Title.
QM 603.F55 1996
612.6'4--dc20   95-52790 CIP

Color reproduction by Colourscan, Singapore
Printed in Italy by A. Mondadori Editore, Verona

To Philippa and Diana
Jack and Rosie

Contents

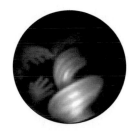
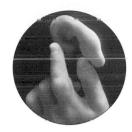
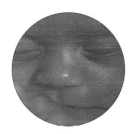
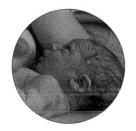

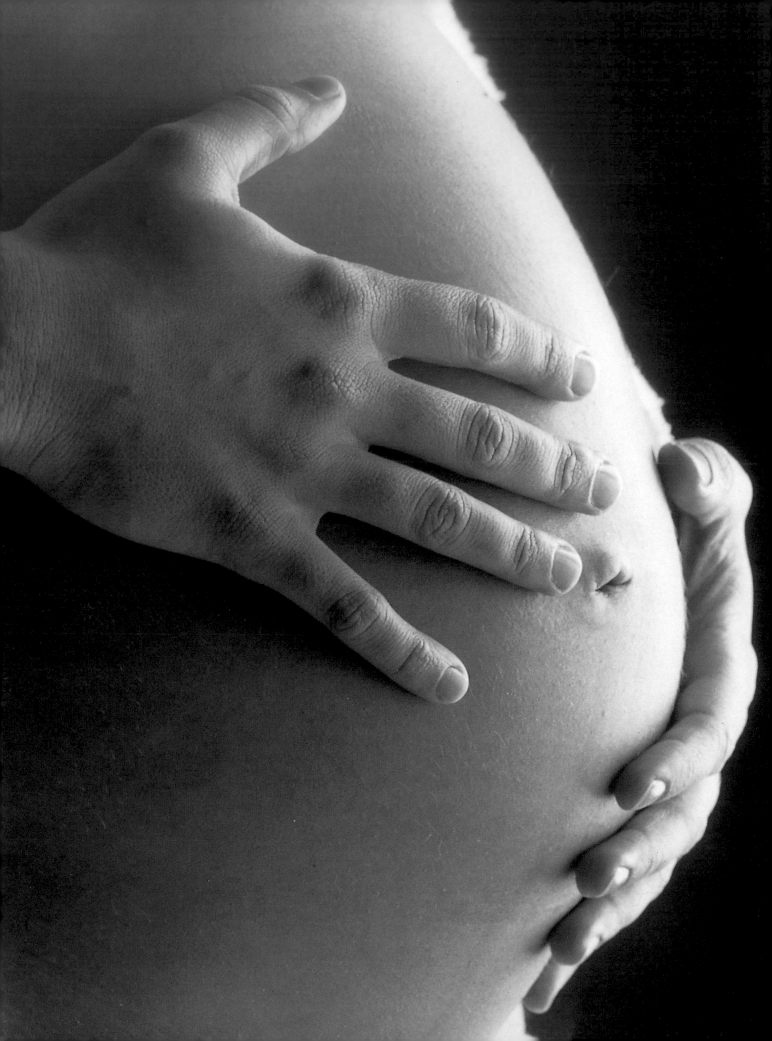

ON THE DAY OF BIRTH this baby will emerge open-eyed, able to see, able to recognize her mother's voice, and also acquainted with the sounds of other voices, with music overheard, and already familiar with all those aspects of the outside world which filter through to her – here, probably a faint glow transmitted from the photographic lights. The womb is not a quiet, isolated place; life within it offers abundant and varied experiences that prepare the baby for the world she will meet when she moves out.

Preface

...those who see things grow from the beginning will have the finest view of them

ARISTOTLE

We are learning to recognize how sensitive, able and already experienced a newly born baby is. She arrives able to breathe and feed, and occasionally can complain loudly. She is also able, in quiet and subtle ways, to respond to people and is so endearing in her actions that she can elicit the loving care she needs. Her competence has developed gradually. New means of observation have made it possible to discover how responsive and active the baby already is in the months preceding birth. Certainly she does not simply lie there curled up in the legendary fetal position.

How can the union of two minutely-small parent cells, egg and sperm, lead to the birth of such an able young person – and in only nine months? Our view of this time, which first shapes all our lives, has become greatly enriched by many specialists, working in different fields of study: ranging from the marvelous microcosm of the cells, to observations of the busy activities of the prenatal baby somersaulting, hearing, touching, tasting. Advanced techniques of photography have often been used in these investigations. I have gathered both pictures and information to weave together the panorama, in words and photographs, from *The first day* to *The day of birth*.

I have drawn on science-based information, relying primarily on what can be carefully observed, measured and recorded. My sources are gratefully acknowledged in the references given on pages 116-117. For the photographs I am grateful to the scientists and medical practitioners who have so generously allowed me to include this important part of their work, acknowledged on page 120.

I have never found this to be "cold science," but colorful and vivid. Out of the great amount of information, I have made my personal choices in selecting those aspects which I myself most enjoyed.

Here and there in this book I have used words such
as "perhaps" and "probably," to allow for individual differences
and to leave open the direction and detail in which our
understanding may develop further. I believe that it will grow
in the direction of seeing our prenatal time as a coherent part
of childhood.

Geraldine Lux Flanagan

Oxford, 1996.

*The age of the baby throughout this book is counted from the day of conception.
In medical practice, prenatal babies are usually dated by "menstrual age," from the
mother's last menstruation, which in effect adds about two weeks to the actual age.*

*Prenatal development for male and female babies is the same, except where specifically
mentioned. So please feel free to substitute "he" for "she," for the baby in this book.*

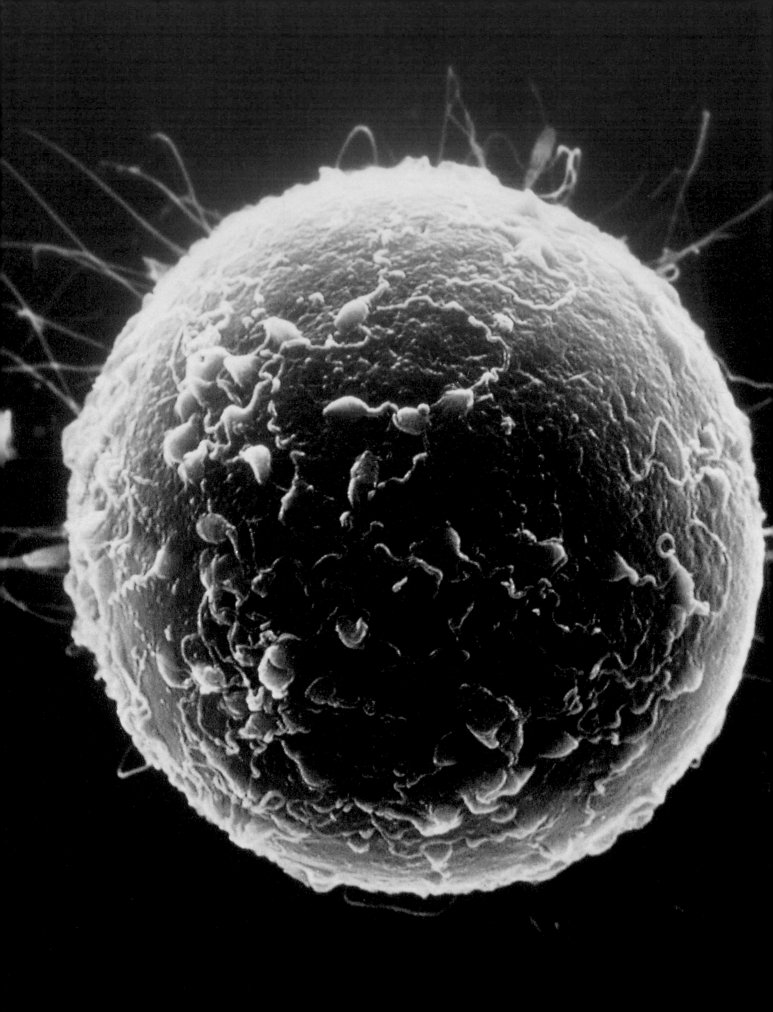

Every baby begins life within

the tiny globe of the mother's egg.

The human egg, here hugely magnified,

is no larger than the dot on this 'i'.

The first day

Before I was born out of my mother generations guided me... WALT WHITMAN

It is beautifully translucent and fragile

and it encompasses the vital links in which

life is carried from one generation to the

next. Within this tiny sphere great events

take place. When one of the father's sperm

A mother's egg magnified 2,000 times with sperm gathered on it, their thin tails standing out. cells, like the ones gathered here around

the egg, succeeds in penetrating the egg and

becomes united with it, a new life can begin.

In the hours of conception every aspect of the genetic inheritance for a new individual will be determined once and for all: to be a boy or girl, with brown, or with blue eyes, fair or dark, tall or short; all the rich detail of physical attributes from head to toes – and also all those complex factors inherited as tendencies, more open to later influences, such as temperament and personality. At the same time, the entry of the one sperm arouses the egg to begin the marvelous process of transforming inert nutrients into a lively being.

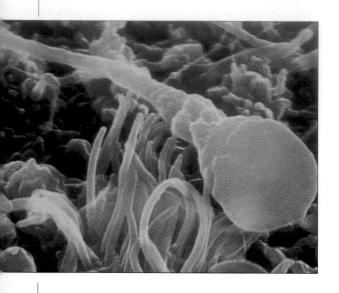

A father's sperm powered by its lashing tail, magnified 9,000 times.

The egg, or *ovum*, comes from the mother's ovary. She may have more than half a million immature eggs stored in her two ovaries. These eggs were formed before the mother's own birth and only a small number of them ever ripens. After puberty only one ovum usually matures each month in alternating ovaries. The ripened egg bursts out and lands in the funnel-shaped opening of the upper end of the fallopian tube. The ovum stays there, immobile and dormant. By itself it probably survives for only a day or two. If it is entered by a sperm during that time, new life is generated; otherwise the egg disintegrates to nothing. Small as it is, the ovum is the largest cell in the human body. In addition to the mother's genetic material the ovum is weighed down by cell substance and is packed with nutrients needed to sustain new life in its first days. Like all eggs the human one too contains some yolk and has a protective outer shell, a soft yet tough membrane called the *zona pellucida* because it is clear and translucent.

Although the cumbersome egg cannot move on its own, it is not powerless. Its presence may attract sperm, perhaps by biochemical signals from the egg's attendant fluids. These signals appear to lead sperm to swim to the egg's vicinity and once there, the egg has the power to excite them and to engage them in attachment and entry.

Far smaller than the egg, the tadpole-shaped sperm cells are among the smallest in the body. They are agile and are good swimmers, able to surge ahead at the rate of about an inch in fifteen minutes, which is an impressive feat for a microscopically small cell. They carry no food, and no freight other than the genetic message from the father together with the means to deliver it. Their power lies in the lashing of their tails and in enzymes around the head of the sperm that can help forge an entry into the egg.

There is a production line of new sperm cells in the father's testicles taking about sixty-four days from start to finish. Usually hundreds of millions of sperm cells are ready, each so small that they would all fit on the head of a thumbtack. Within the man's body they can remain alive and immobilized for several weeks. They suddenly become active when, at ejaculation, perhaps two hundred million sperm are swept out on a tide of semen. In a mere droplet there may be a quarter of a million or even a million sperm cells. But they are not all alike; at least a third of them appear to be oddly formed and not very good

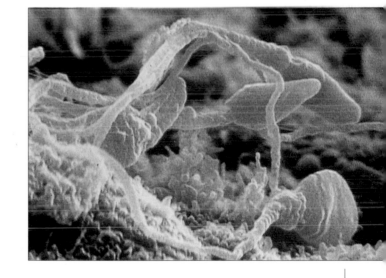

Out of a tide of millions
some surge ahead, some lag behind.
These sperm are seen in a fallopian tube
through a scanning electron microscope.

▷ *Egg-getters' phalanx starting in formation. Each dot here is a sperm.*

at swimming. Until recently these have been classified as defective but now there is evidence that they might be a group of so-called "kamikaze" sperm. Their brief role in life may be to lag behind and, in effect, occupy the entrance against any possible rival father's sperm while the vigorous "egg-getters" charge ahead. In the words of Aldous Huxley:

A million million spermatozoa,

All of them alive:

Out of their cataclysm but one poor Noah

Dare hope to survive.

The egg-getters must make an approximately seven-inch journey, first through the cervix, then on through the small cavern of the uterus, and then into the correct one of the two hair-fine openings of the fallopian tubes, and finally on up to its far end. The egg-getters start in a phalanx and further on disperse "like scouting parties looking for an egg." Some go astray and most of them perish on the way, so that only several dozen of the fittest, or luckiest, out of the starting millions will reach the goal. When no egg is waiting, the sperm survivors can hang on at rest with their heads clinging to the wall of the fallopian tube. They can survive like that for several days. Since egg and sperm can each await the other, this stretches the time around ovulation during which a baby may be conceived – nature ever enhancing the likelihood of this event.

Sperm can wait *hanging on for several days in the channel to the egg.*

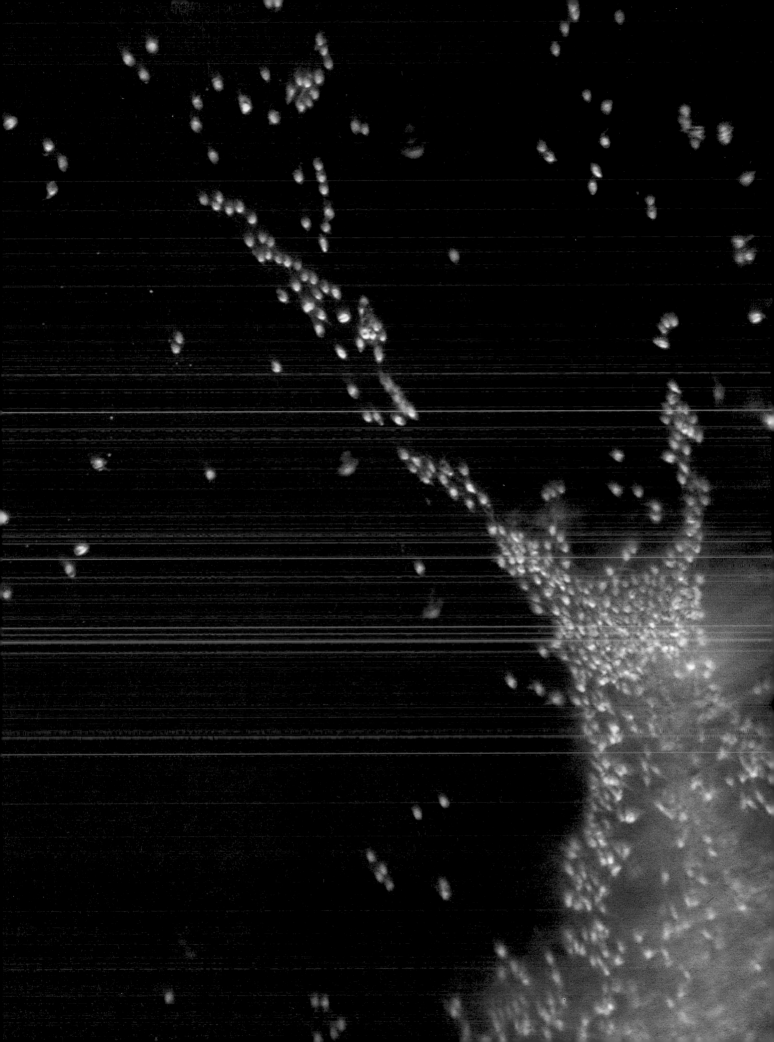

The event is further helped along under the influence of the hormones accompanying ovulation and may be boosted by sexual arousal. On ovulation, waves of contractions are set in motion in the walls of the fallopian tubes, and perhaps also in the uterus, creating an upward current of fluids toward the place where the egg is parked. And so the sperm-cell swimmers may be speeded on their way to make the seven-inch crossing in less than half an hour! Even the stragglers usually get there in three to four hours.

But they could not get there at all, were it not for another hormonal response within the mother's body. The entrance to her uterus is normally filled with protective mucus, the cervical mucus composed of sugars and proteins. Most of the time, this mucus is so thick that sperm can hardly traverse it. They become entangled in it.

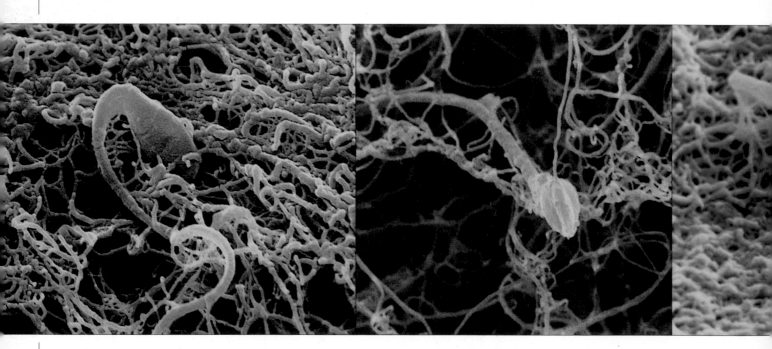

Sperm entangled
in the mucus thicket which normally
guards the entrance to the womb.

Navigating elegantly
a sperm is swimming through the widened gaps
in the mucus maze at the time of ovulation.

As you can see under great magnification, the mucus is made up of a thicket of netlike strands. It is like a dense hedge that guards the entryway into the uterus. However, around the time of ovulation the mucus becomes watery. This loosens the net and sperm can navigate through the gaps. Sperm must be able to make their way across this obstacle course under their own steam and many fail. Only the best of the egg-getters succeed in their zigzag course through the maze and reach the next stage, from where they may have a speedy ascent, aided by the current of maternal fluids.

The buoyant immersion in the maternal fluids not only provides transport, it has another vital function. The exposure to fallopian-tube fluids appears to be essential for sperm to become potent and capable of penetrating and fertilizing an egg. As they travel along, sperm become "capacitated" on the way, prepared and ready for an encounter with the egg. If an egg is waiting, the sperm cells are ready to respond.

Such is the power of the egg that the sperm finalists become visibly excited when they reach the egg's vicinity, so excited that they are described as being hyperactivated. Each sperm cell has its own mode of showing it. The individual swimming styles of their hyperactive final lap have been

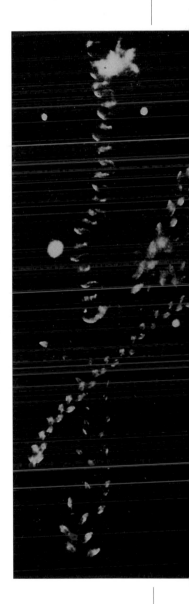

Zigzag tracks
record the swimming
styles of sperm
crossing the mucus.

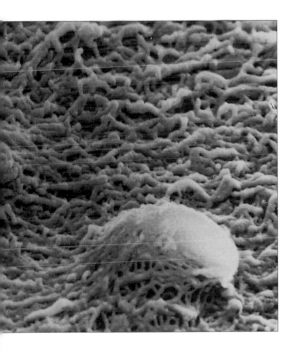

Totally trapped
sperm is caught in the much denser
mucus in the later months of pregnancy.

given the colorful names of "thrash," "wide-amplitude," and the intriguing "star-spin." By thrash, star-spin, or wide-amplitude, the surviving horde vigorously homes in around the egg.

Once in contact, sperm and egg recognize each other in a biological sense by the exact fit of the molecules on their mutual surfaces. The close-fit molecules interlock and the sperm cells become fastened to the soft shell of the egg, its *zona pellucida*. The mere two or three dozen sperm cells to have succeeded this far are now acted upon by a special protein contained within the zona. In response, each sperm cell sheds its own outer covering, which has been like a cap over its head. The lifting of its head cap exposes the sperm's special enzymes. These can dissolve a microscopic slit in the egg's zona but perhaps only if the sperm has hit upon a favorable entry-site. A hyperactivated sperm cell can then struggle through to enter the egg.

Homing in hyperactive sperm compete to penetrate the egg's shell, here hugely magnified.

This becomes a competition: which one will be first? Each carries its own genetic program and each is different from the rest in uncountable details, including whether the child will be a boy or girl. The father's sperm alone carries the genetic message to dictate the gender of the baby, and the sex will be decided when one sperm manages to penetrate the egg just ahead of the others. That sperm cell will be instantly zipped into the egg, tail and all. This is the moment of fertilization. There is an immediate reaction in the egg. All the other sperm contenders are shut out and the egg ceases to be available to later sperm arrivals. The female egg seems most monogamous.

The egg is dramatically aroused from its dormant state upon the entry of the one successful sperm. Many aspects of this spark of life are a mystery. We know only that the egg's biological machinery

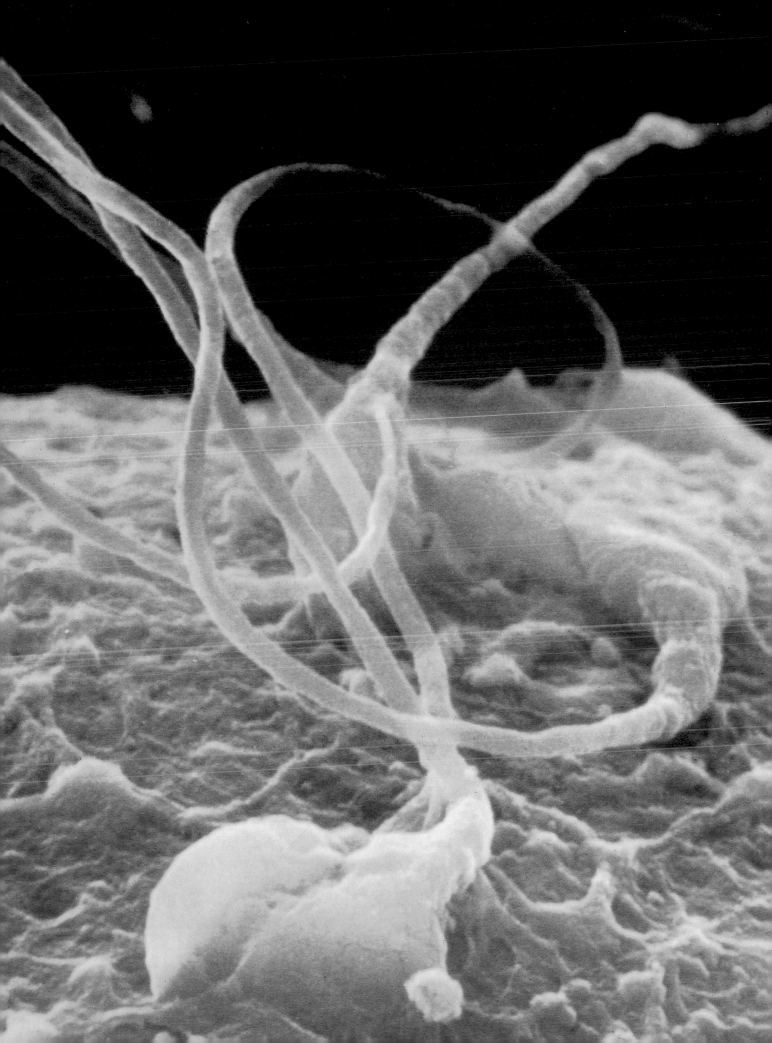

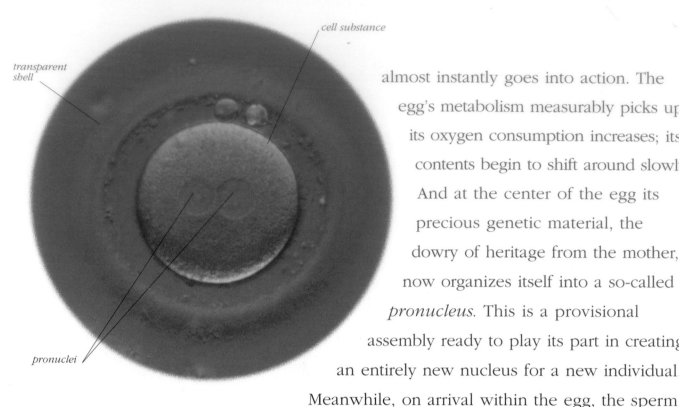

transparent
shell

cell substance

pronuclei

*Parents' pronuclei
lie side by side in
the egg. Its fragile
transparency is
revealed by
microscope light.*

almost instantly goes into action. The egg's metabolism measurably picks up; its oxygen consumption increases; its contents begin to shift around slowly. And at the center of the egg its precious genetic material, the dowry of heritage from the mother, now organizes itself into a so-called *pronucleus*. This is a provisional assembly ready to play its part in creating an entirely new nucleus for a new individual.

Meanwhile, on arrival within the egg, the sperm has shed its tail and has rested for a few hours. Then the tailless sperm head, filled with the father's genetic dowry, wanders very slowly toward the center of the egg. There, it gradually swells up and organizes itself into the paternal pronucleus, a complete match in size and importance for the maternal one.

In each pronucleus there are twenty-three pairs of strands called *chromosomes*. These are visible only under a microscope. Arranged on these chromosomes are the very much smaller genes. No one as yet knows their exact number; they are now being counted in the course of the Human Genome Project. It is estimated that as many as one hundred thousand genes may be carried in our chromosomes, one half of these coming from each parent, contributed in the parental pronucleus. The genes consist of the substance known as DNA. Imagined as a molecular alphabet, the DNA spells out what is to be: first of all to be human in design and function, more specifically to be a member of this family, to follow what has been genetically passed down the line by all previous generations. But with as many as a hundred thousand paired parental genes in play there are vast possibilities for new combinations of the ancestral genes. The result is bound to be different from any ancestor. It will be an entirely new genetic program for a unique new individual.

The new genetic program is achieved when the two parent pronuclei come to lie side by side within the egg for perhaps a day, as their contents combine in the ultimate biological union of male and female. In the instant when the union is consummated, the whole egg substance divides into two entirely new cells, identical to one another. These are the first two cells of the baby-to-be. So begins the first day of the first nine months of life.

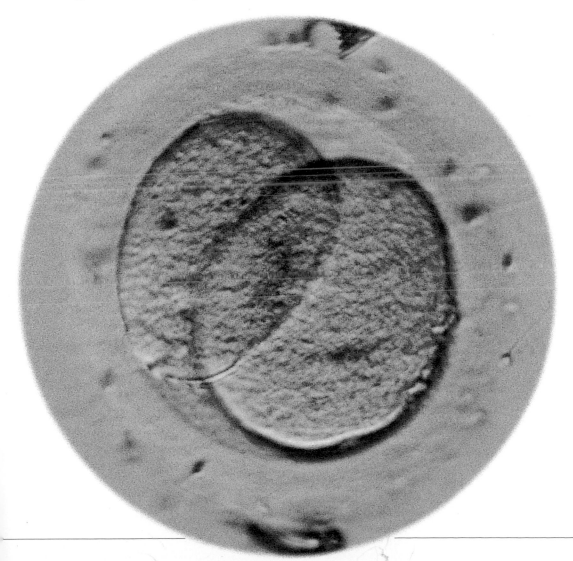

The first two cells of the baby-to-be within the egg's translucent shell.

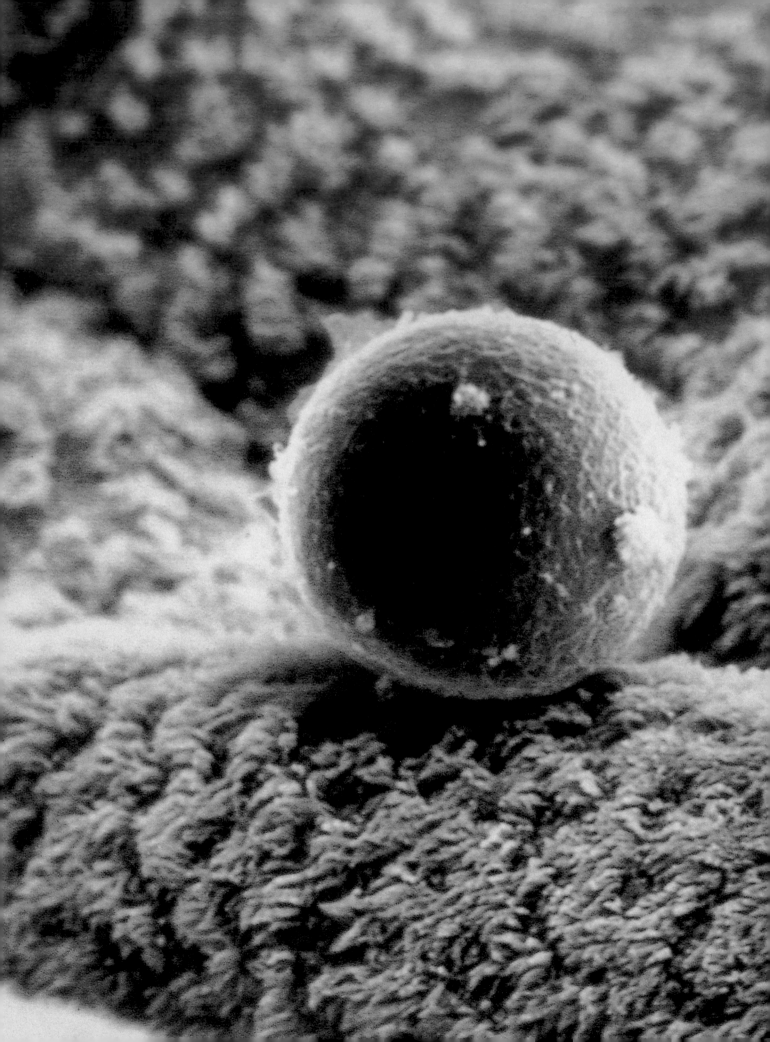

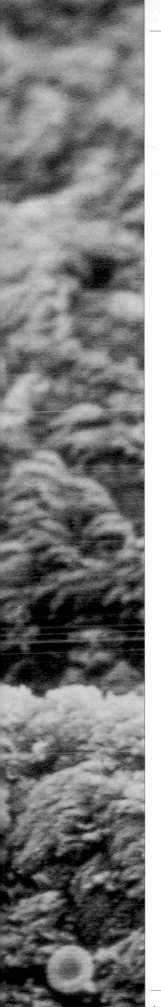

Day by day the first two cells of the new life steadily divide and subdivide, about once in every twenty-four hours, and so

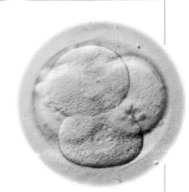

Four cells

The first week

Your children are ... life's longing for itself KHALIL GIBRAN

generate a cluster of four, then eight, then sixteen and by the end of this week already well over a hundred cells. During this time, the tiny sphere of cells, with defeated sperm cells still clinging to its surface, drifts slowly downstream and toward the womb.

The sphere
*drifts downstream. Within
the shell, dividing cells
(above, right) are illuminated.*

25

After their arrival in the uterus the new cells will hatch; they will emerge from their protective zona shell. Then, on about the seventh day, the hatched cells will begin to nest in the mother's nourishing tissues, to be embedded there until birth.

On the way to the womb the delicate new cells can survive only in a watery environment. Indeed, under great magnification the scene within the channel of the fallopian tube looks like an underwater ocean landscape. This is a sort of sea within the mother, provided through evolution. It cushions the developing cells, keeps them from

A "sea within" the fluid-filled maternal channel with its sweeping lashes, magnified 30,000 times.

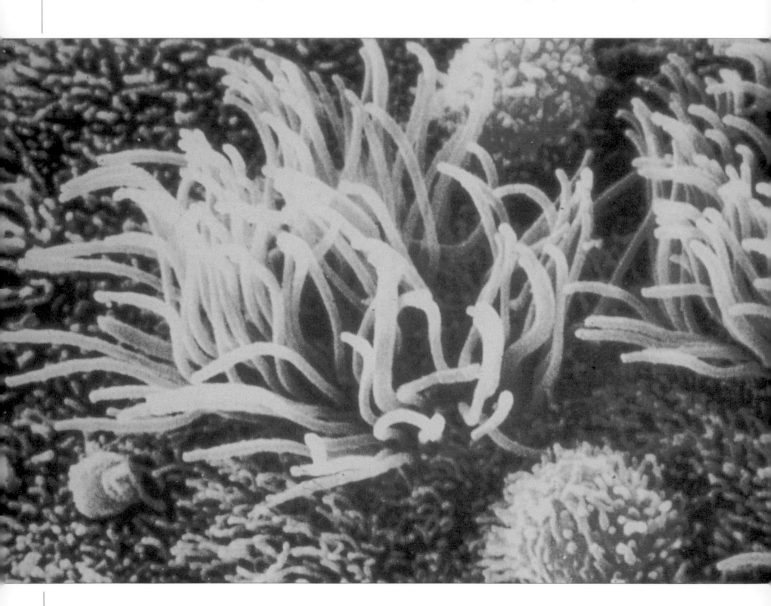

dehydration, maintains an even temperature, provides salts and sugars
as slight nourishment that the cells absorb, and also contains substances
that prepare the cluster for its nesting. At the same time, the fluids
lend the transport needed to convey the cluster to its nesting site.

The cluster travels like flotsam. It is wafted along by the
currents within the fallopian tube. But the stream that sped
the swimming sperm out to the waiting egg has now completely
reversed its flow. This happens because the wavelike contractions,
and the brushlike sweeping by *cilia* (meaning lashes), within the

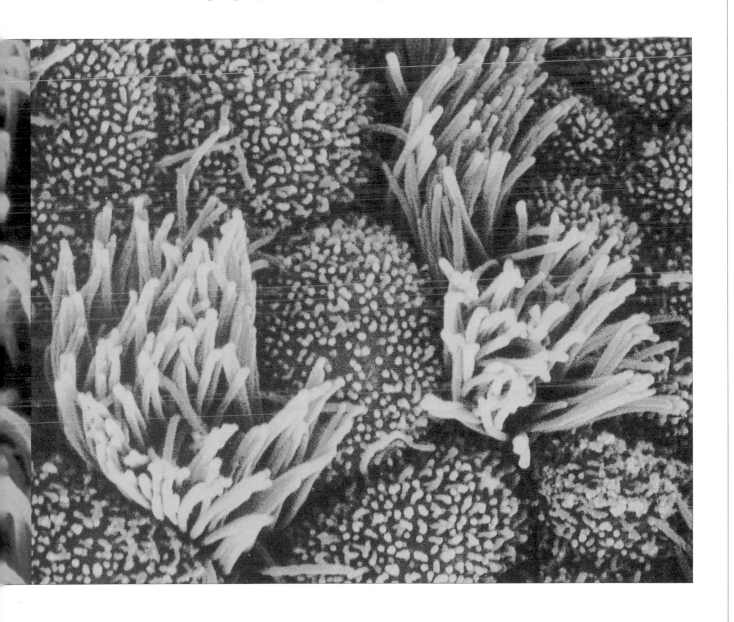

walls of the fallopian tube have switched direction. The current now goes toward the uterus. The remarkable reversal of this flow is in direct response to changing maternal hormones. Although the cluster is free-floating, it transmits an almost immediate biochemical signal, an "I am here" message. Within about twenty-four hours of being fertilized, the new cells begin to produce minute but increasing amounts of a hormone called hCG, short for human Chorionic Gonadotrophin. This hormone is released into the bloodstream of the mother where it can be detected by the end of this week by a special blood test as the earliest sign of pregnancy. A week later it shows up in the standard home pregnancy test. The presence of hCG leads to the production of a key hormone in the mother's ovary.

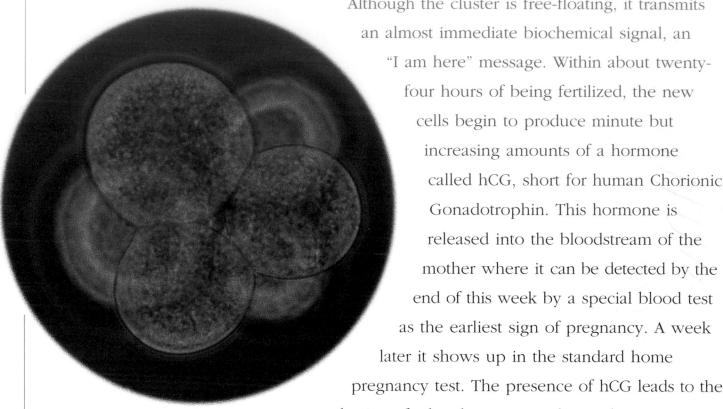

"I am here:"
six to eight cells
by day 3 transmit
a signal.

That hormone forestalls the next menstruation, and altogether starts to make the mother's body hospitable for the nesting embryo-to-be. Thus the new life contributes to creating a mother for itself.

The cluster's journey down the fallopian tube lasts three to four days. During this time the cells increase to about a dozen or perhaps sixteen. It is not an entirely predictable nor always an even number, because some single cells may fail and die off without harm to the healthy development of the rest. From the beginning cell death is part of life. But quite often all may fail. It is probably nature's "fail-safe" if the early cell divisions have gone awry, or other conditions are not

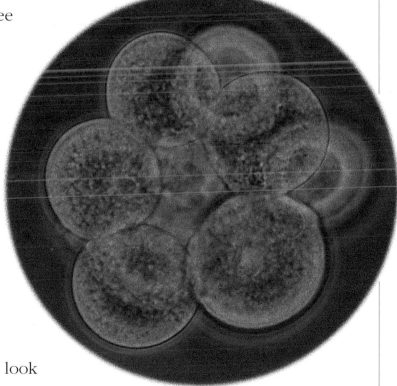

favorable on this occasion. It is estimated that more than half of incipient pregnancies may end here, many of them too early to have been recognized. The cluster, small as the smallest particle of dust, disappears unnoticed.

◁ An early portrait of their offspring for IVF parents.

This is a precarious time. But the first days are also the best time to transfer into the mother an egg fertilized *in vitro*, meaning "in glass," in a medical laboratory. The transfer is usually made after the cluster has reached four to eight cells. In the laboratory one can watch through a microsope how these cells divide and IVF parents can have a really early photograph of their offspring. It is wonderful to see these translucent, fragile-looking first cells in motion as each slowly, very slowly, draws itself in across its middle and then suddenly, there are two cells where there was one. Here the cells look like grainy bubbles. Under greater magnification one would see that they are not empty. Each contains a nucleus which, in turn, contains the chromosomes holding the new genetic program for this person. In addition each cell contains a complex of fine filaments and structures, the biological machinery that carries out the genetic program and passes it on from cell to cell.

The "mulberry" ten cells, later on day 3, bathed in pink IVF nutrient.

The early cells are closely bunched together and are named *morula*, meaning "mulberry," because when magnified they look somewhat like one. While the "mulberry" is traveling toward the uterus, it reaches between a dozen to sixteen cells that are, as far as we know, identical to one another. If, as rarely but regularly happens, these identical cells separate themselves into two or more lots, this will lead to identical twins or triplets or more. All these begin their parallel development at this early stage or within the next few days.

The minute mulberry cluster enters the uterus on about its fourth day. There the cluster drifts around for two or three more days while the cell numbers steadily double and redouble, and mount to over a hundred. Since the cells increase in number by dividing themselves, the individual ones become smaller and smaller, and their total volume does not increase. Therefore the entire cluster can still be contained within the slightly stretched zona shell of the

Eight to ten cells *are transparent and transmit the background color; shut-out sperm still cruise around the zona shell.*

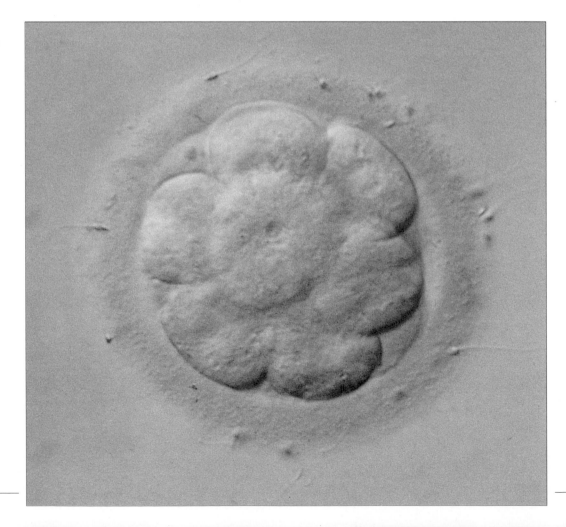

original egg. The zona prevents the cluster from becoming attached too soon. This was particularly advantageous on the way through the fallopian tube because it protected the cluster, and also the mother, from the mutual dangers of implantation in that narrow channel.

While the unattached cluster floats over the surface of the uterus a major change happens: the cells cease to be identical. They become significantly different from one another. As they become differentiated they arrange themselves into two distinct groupings, an inner and an outer one.

Inner and outer cells will have vitally different destinies. The inner cell mass will give rise to the embryo, leading on to the baby and in time the adult – leading to all the cells of this individual's life time. The outer group of cells will have a

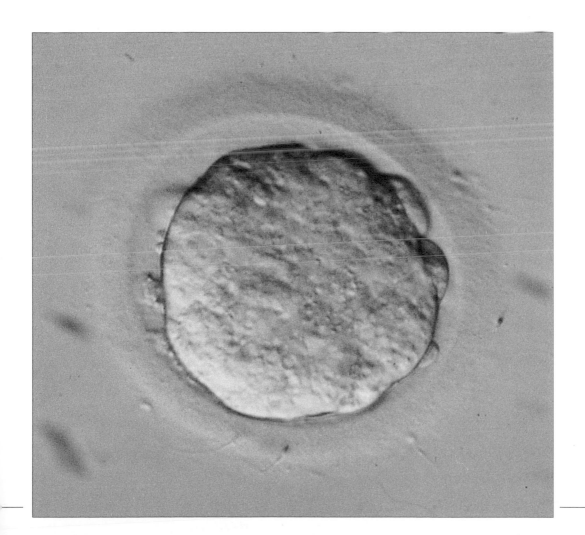

Sixteen cells by day 4, tightly packed within the zona, still no larger than the dot on this 'i'.

relatively brief life, lasting for only the nine months until birth. These outer cells, perhaps garnering a few inner ones, will give rise to a temporary support system: all the vessels and structures including the placenta, or afterbirth, dedicated to nourishing, housing, and protecting the baby before birth. At birth these tissues will have outlived their function and will be discarded. It is not known what determines the initial assignment to the inner or outer group. It may be like musical chairs, just the chance of where a cell happens to be

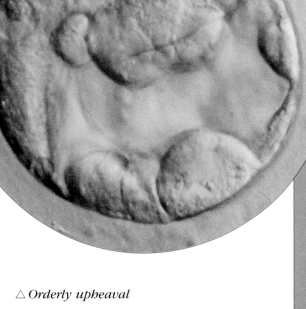

△ *Orderly upheaval*
as the cells rearrange
themselves into an inner
and an outer group with
differing destinies.

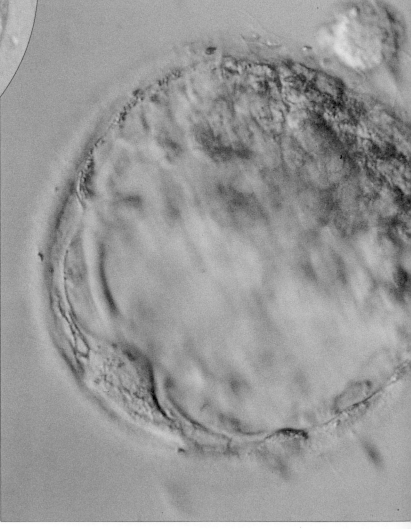

placed when differentiation begins. The differentiated cells go on increasing their numbers, and continuously arrange and rearrange themselves in a highly organized way. They become a *blastocyst*, meaning "sprout pouch." The young sprout is ready to hatch, as this step is rightly called: the zona shell gives way, the cells ooze out. When the newly hatched cells come in contact with the surface of the uterus they can begin to attach themselves.

Now the cluster is ready to settle down. Usually this will be within the upper curve of the uterus, the place most likely to lead to an uncomplicated birth nine months hence. How does the cluster make such an astonishingly "forward-looking" selection?

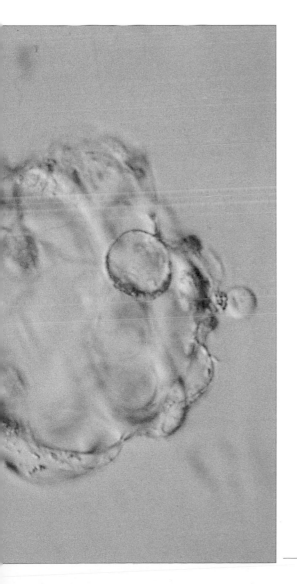

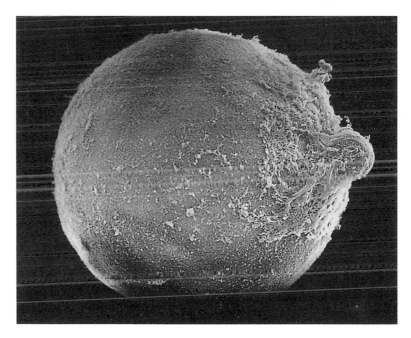

Hatching

the shell gives way, the cells poke out:
this moment is caught by an electron
microscope (above). Then, seen through
an ordinary microscope (left) the mass of
new cells oozes out from the round shell.

We do not know; it remains a puzzle. The spot for settling will most likely also offer the advantage of proximity to useful maternal blood vessels offering ready access to nourishment.

On about the seventh day, the newly hatched cells start to nest. They burrow into the lining of the uterus. Since the nesting cells are genetically different from the mother it has long been another puzzle that they are not rejected, as a transplant or graft would be. Even donor eggs would be accepted. The answer turns out to be that the cell cluster suppresses its genetic markers and instead gives out special signals that can be compared to a universal password. The password is the same for all people and is the same one that the mother's cells expressed when she herself was just such a cluster. Therefore, her cells do not now mobilize defenses against the new arrivals because they biologically recognize the nesting cluster as universal friend not foe.

The womb accepts the friendly invader. The nesting cells soon develop outshoots of fine *villi*, meaning "tufts of hair." Like roots, the villi will aid in absorbing nutrients from the mother's blood circulation, just as a plant absorbs nourishment from wet soil. In addition to gathering nourishment, the villi also serve to implant the cells securely.

By the end of the first week the invaded maternal tissue heals over and covers the nesting cells with a capsule that gives them extra protection and anchoring. Within the opaque walls of this dome a spectacular metamorphosis will take place. Soon the cluster of cells, increasing and changing every hour, will be transformed into a distinctly human embryo with head and body, arms and legs, and even fingers and toes.

Nesting
the friendly invader settles into the lining of the uterus under a sheltering dome of maternal tissue.

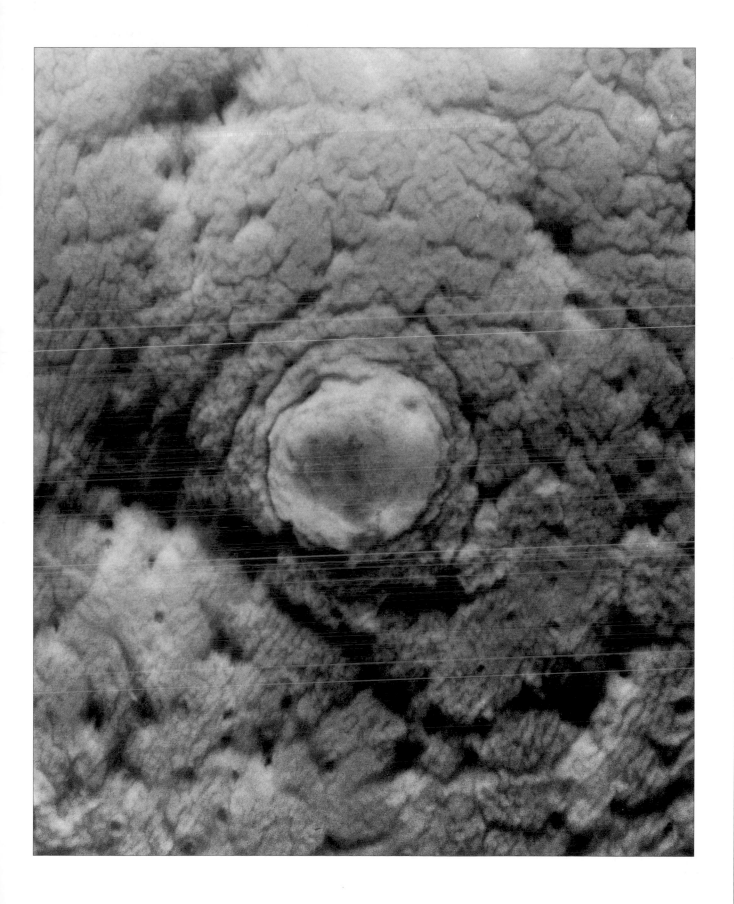

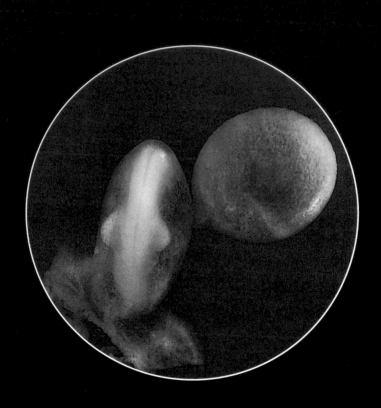

Life-size

This one month will bring a marvelous transformation, the greatest developmental change of a lifetime. The hundreds of cells turn into many thousands and together they become ten thousand times larger than the early cluster had been.

The first month

...no one who studies development can fail to be filled with a sense of wonder and delight.

LEWIS WOLPERT: *The Triumph of the Embryo*

A tiny body at four weeks: a large head, curved back, and arm buds. Its 'balloon' is where blood cells are made.

The wonder of it is that these myriad cells organize themselves into a human body with the beginnings of all its exquisitely specialized components, all in their right places and some already practicing their functions.

In the fourth week, the tiny heart will begin to beat regularly, pumping a trickle of newly formed blood through minute blood vessels; the rudimentary brain will already show human specialization; the kidneys will prepare to produce droplets of urine; the arm buds will form, followed by leg buds, and in the next month the limbs will start to move. And all along, the face molds itself with beginnings for eyes, ears, nose, and mouth. Everything is still very small and primitive. Even after the vast increase in size by the end of this month, the whole body is only about a quarter of an inch, merely six millimeters long, as at the top corner of the preceding page.

The cluster of cells has become an *embryo*, which means to "teem within." If we could watch this body-building process under magnification we would indeed see a teeming traffic of cells. Great cell migrations streaming along in groups, reaching their various destinations and piling up, building folds which then unfurl, forming organs, molding features; cells ever dividing and increasing their numbers, taking on new shapes and becoming specialized to be brain or heart or liver or lung or arm or eye. A multitude of many different kinds of cells will be needed for all the structural and functioning parts of the baby. And more: the baby will need its own life-support system in the uterus, including the placenta and umbilical cord. Groups of teeming cells become dedicated to establishing all this as well.

The organization for the body began in the very first week when the nesting cluster's embryo-making cells distinguished themselves from life-support cells. In the second week, when there are many more cells, sheets of embryo-making cells stream along to form three layers. One will go on to be brain, spinal cord, nerves and skin; the second to be digestive system, liver and pancreas; the third layer to be heart, blood vessels, muscles, and skeleton. It is a busy scene yet so orderly that, given some leeway for individual variation, we can draw up a daily diary of development.

On about the ninth day the cell layers arrange themselves into the embryonic shield, so-called because it has the shape of a shield under the microscope. Its broad top maps out where the embryo's head will be, the narrow tip appoints the bottom. Within this shield, cells amass in a central streak marking out the midline of the body. All along this streak cells continue to pile up until there are enough of them to fold over and form a tube. This is the beginning of the all-important neural tube. It is the foundation for the brain and the nervous system. From here cells build forward to assemble the two lobes for the brain, which gets a headstart in development. This will give the embryo a big head and gives the brain maximum time for development. As the lobes for the brain progress in the third week, the body elongates and is so delicately transparent that the foundation for the neural tube and spinal column is plain to see.

These delicate tissues need to be in protective fluid and the

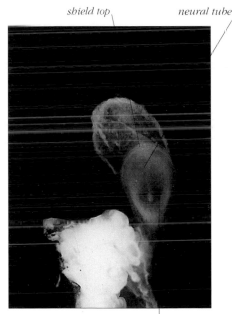

shield top *neural tube*

shield bottom

Embryonic shield
in week 2: teeming cells establish where head, bottom, and neural tube will be.

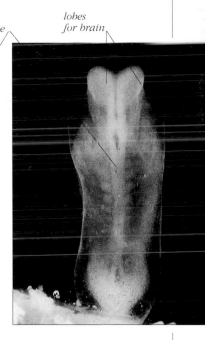

lobes for brain

Headstart
in week 3: body, neural tube, and two lobes for brain have advanced.

accompanying support-system cells provide for this. By the fourth week, they have formed a membrane which resembles a fluid-filled bubble surrounding the embryo. The cluster of cells has given way to the very small figure, seen on page 36, with budding arms, with its back gently curved and its large head leaning forwards.

The tiny embryo needs its own blood circulation to distribute nutrients and oxygen all around the fast-growing territory of cells. The embryo is not like a machine, first made and then made to go. It is a working organism from the start, and on each day has to be fit to survive on that day and also be ready for the demands of the next day's expansion of its business. And so, back on about day 13, well in advance of the needed circulation, a group of cells moves into position where the chest will be. These cells arrange themselves into a U-shaped tube to become the heart. Simultaneously, other cells start to form a circuit of tubular vessels, extending all around the body. In perfect coordination, the production of cells for blood is initiated to fill these vessels. In only eight or nine days, by about day 21 or 22, the primitive heart tube begins to twitch, and by about day 25 the heart gets into its stride to beat regularly, never to stop for this lifetime. As the heart starts to beat, the embryo's own blood is ready and comes coursing in. By the fourth week it is pumped through the new circuit of blood vessels and continuously travels all around the developing body, delivering nutrients and oxygen, and picking up wastes from all the working cells.

The wellspring of provisions for the embryo is the mother's blood supply. The embryo can get what it needs because some of the cells of the original cluster moved outward to establish supply lines for the embryo's complex support system. The first week's rootlike villi develop into a profuse branching network embedded in the wall of the womb. These villi can draw sufficient nourishment for the embryo's immediate requirements. But the embryo will soon need more, and the villi gradually become incorporated into a much more elaborate supply system that will develop fully in the next two months. But even now, the support system is larger, and weighs more, than the embryo itself. The linking umbilical cord will be an essential part of the supply lines. By the third week the cord is started, still primitive but a good enough conduit for the modest flow of blood pumped by the embryo's newly beating heart.

Development is so forward-looking that in establishing the embryo there is already provision for the next generation. The special cells to generate the eggs or sperm that this new girl or boy will carry are differentiated now and migrate to the newly forming reproductive organs.

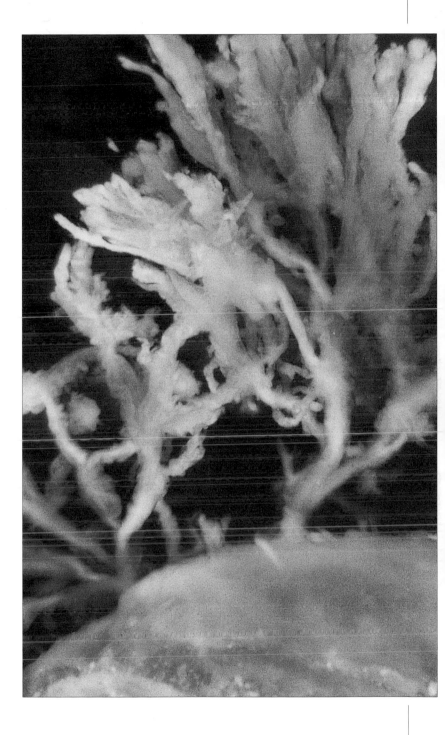

Branches of villi similar to fine roots, they carry sustenance to the embryo. Here 17 times enlarged.

How is such far-reaching organization achieved? What makes the cells act as if they know where to go, and what to be, and what to do when they get there? And also act in such harmony with their fellow cells? These big questions take us into the world of the almost infinitesimally small molecules within the cells, primarily those that compose the genes and make up the genetic program. Since the advent of molecular biology it is for the first time becoming possible to detect and describe some of these processes. "Life's book, it seemed, was suddenly laid open…," although only some fascinating pages of it. We are still far from understanding the whole story.

It is clear that cells work together so well because there is a continual molecular dialogue between them and they adapt their intrinsic genetic instructions accordingly. The instructions are held in the genes in the form of the so-called genetic code, spelled out in the arrangement of molecules, like letters of a special alphabet. The genetic program for the baby, spelled out in that code, was achieved on the first day in the union of parent cells. From then on, every time any cell divided and gave rise to two new cells, a precise replica of all the genes was made and passed along to each new cell. Therefore every cell of the body carries exactly the same genes, and holds the full genetic program.

Every cell might simply go on to produce clones of itself, all with the same destination and function, if the full program were to be active all the time. What makes for the great variety of cells produced, and for their dispersal to all their different destinations, is the fact that genes can switch on and switch off. Not all of them are operative all the time. This happens in response to signals from fellow cells as they all fit themselves into the elaborate program of development.

These events may be visualized as if the cells were a large group of participants engaged in an exacting building task requiring close cooperation. Each knows the grand plan, each gives out signals, and in turn sensitively responds to the signals from others to become integrated into the whole project. The cells of the embryo work in a comparable way, in companionable agreement, with genes switched on and off as required.

In setting the overall program there appears to be a hierarchy of functions within the genes. Among the genes high up in the hierarchy there are some surprising ones, which have been given the homely name of *Homeobox,* or *Hox* for short. The Hox genes contain even more domestic-sounding regions called *homeodomains.* The wonderful and surprising aspect of these gene domains is that we share them with other forms of life, with other animals and even plants. The homeodomains are thought to be "conserved," that is, genetic information has been passed on intact, not only from parent to child but also from one form of life to another, through billions of years of evolution. And so we all carry that historic record within us and in this way all of life on earth is truly related.

The conserved homeodomains are thought to have a fundamental role in giving the general architectural plan, and all cells carry this coded information: start from one cell, build a bunch of cells, the head goes here, the bottom there, and so on. It is thought that there may be further conserved genes for other kinds of genetic "know-how" on, for instance, how to fashion an eye.

As a cell becomes dedicated to a particular place and

46 chromosomes *the genetic program for a baby is packaged in these strands. Every new cell carries exact copies of all 46.*

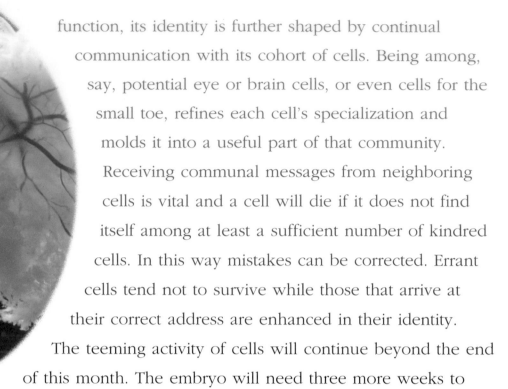

The embryo encircled by its lacy villi. Communities of cells have established all its working parts.

function, its identity is further shaped by continual communication with its cohort of cells. Being among, say, potential eye or brain cells, or even cells for the small toe, refines each cell's specialization and molds it into a useful part of that community. Receiving communal messages from neighboring cells is vital and a cell will die if it does not find itself among at least a sufficient number of kindred cells. In this way mistakes can be corrected. Errant cells tend not to survive while those that arrive at their correct address are enhanced in their identity.

The teeming activity of cells will continue beyond the end of this month. The embryo will need three more weeks to have a complete body. Improvements come quickly. On about day 24, the embryo does not yet have any visible arms but within two days, on about day 26, the budding arms assemble as simple knobs at the sides of the body. Within only about forty-eight hours, there already will be demarcations for upper and lower arms. And the budding legs will follow a few days later. Next month, the limbs will lengthen, hands and fingers, feet and toes will develop, and the embryo will begin to move them, and wiggle and turn its whole body as it bobs about in its fluid-filled bubble.

Heading into next month the embryo, here seen from behind, will soon be able to move by itself.

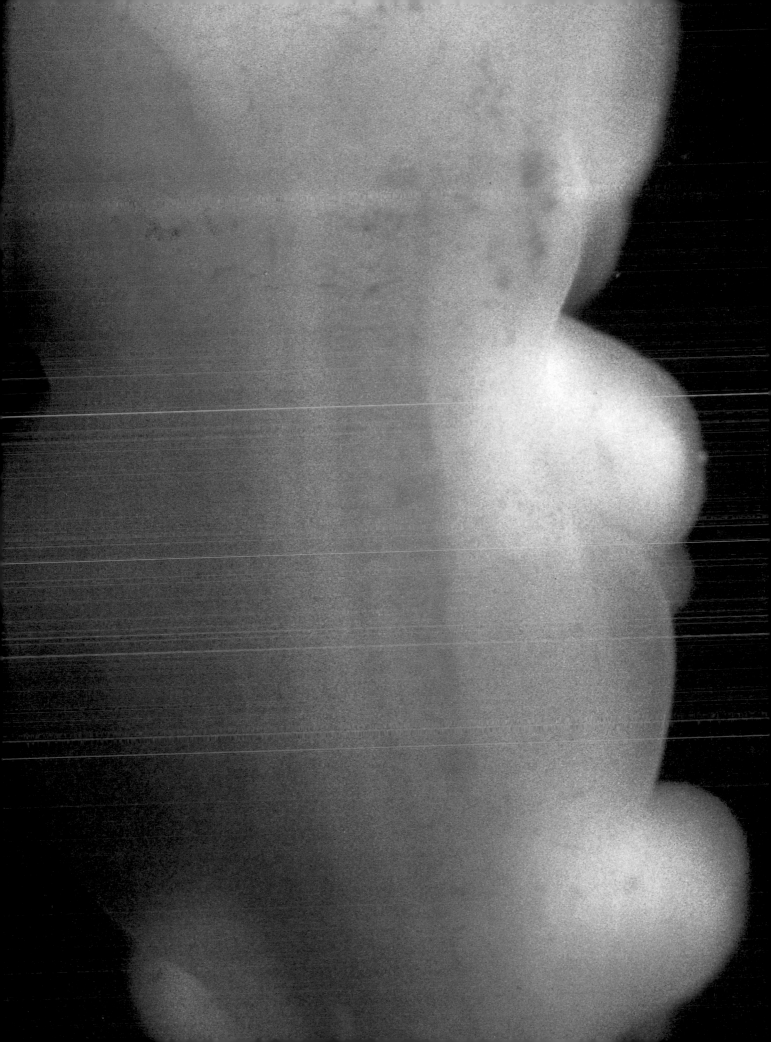

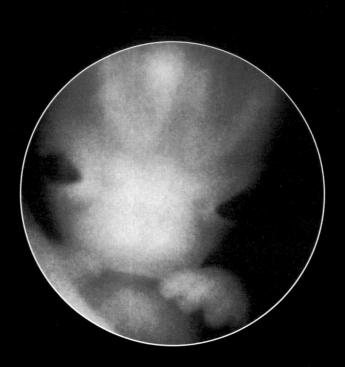

A gentle face with open eyes greets us in the seventh week, photographed by a miniature camera looking into the womb. The embryo's hands touch the face with stubby fingers; the high forehead is testimony to the prominent human brain.

The second month

...a cell which has as all its progeny the human brain. The mere existence of such a cell should be one of the great astonishments of this earth. LEWIS THOMAS

A gentle face meets a camera in the womb in the seventh week.

The first three weeks of this month lead to the completion of the body as the primitive embryo develops into a small-scale baby, only about one inch in height, and so light and delicate that it weighs no more than one whole peanut.

Yet at seven weeks this tiny being will have, in miniature, the foundations for all the organs and structures needed even for the future adult. There is provision for everything, down to such details as tooth buds in the gums, taste buds on the tongue, beds for finger-nails, and also the foundations for reproductive and sexual organs. From then on there will be mainly a great increase in size and weight, a change in proportions, and many refinements in structure and function. But even before the primitive body is completed it is increasingly functioning: the brain begins to produce some measurable impulses, the kidneys extract waste and put out urine, the liver takes over production of blood cells, the stomach produces digestive juices, and the heart is pumping sturdily, beating

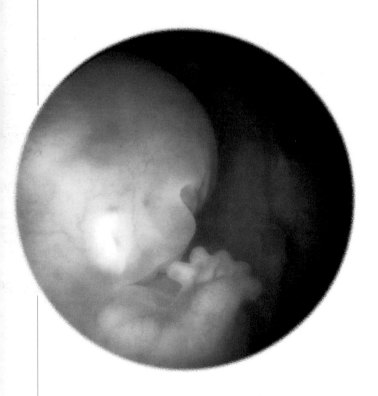

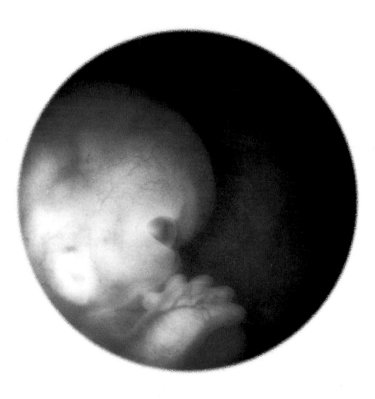

The embryo
afloat in its home environment in the womb, disclosed within the circular aperture of an endoscopic camera. The embryo's stubby fingers touch around the mouth.

One inch tall
in sitting height; the embryo's eyes are unfinished, their lids still to grow; the extended thumb will invite sucking soon. The placenta is in the background (opposite page).

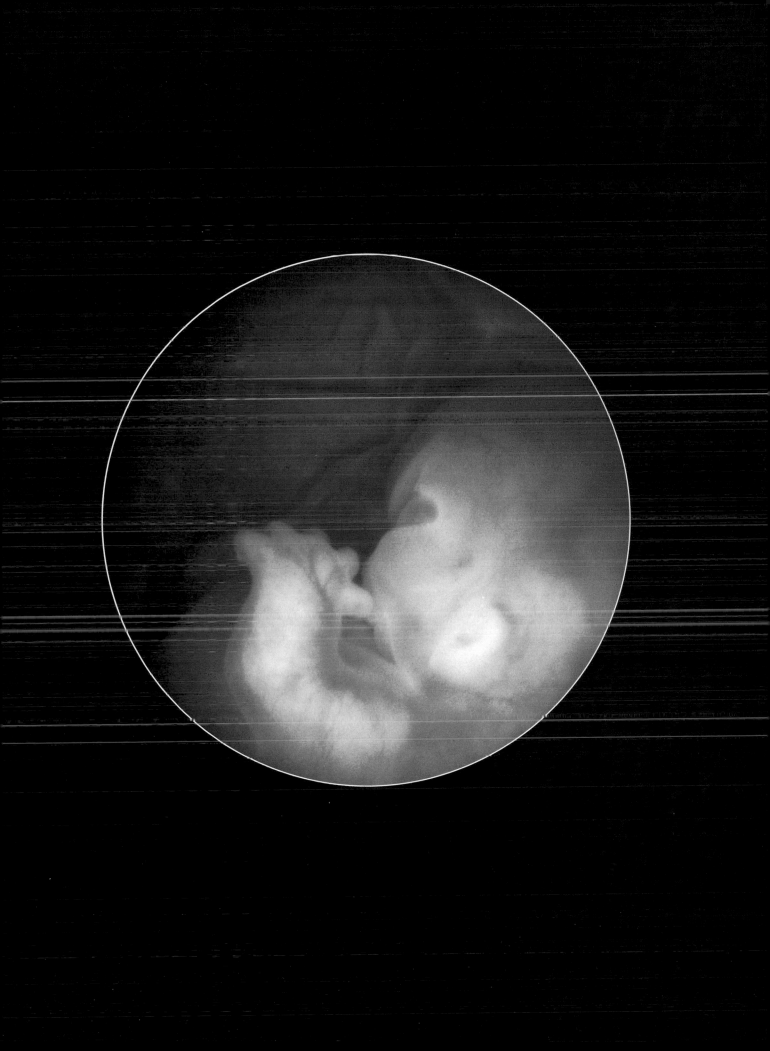

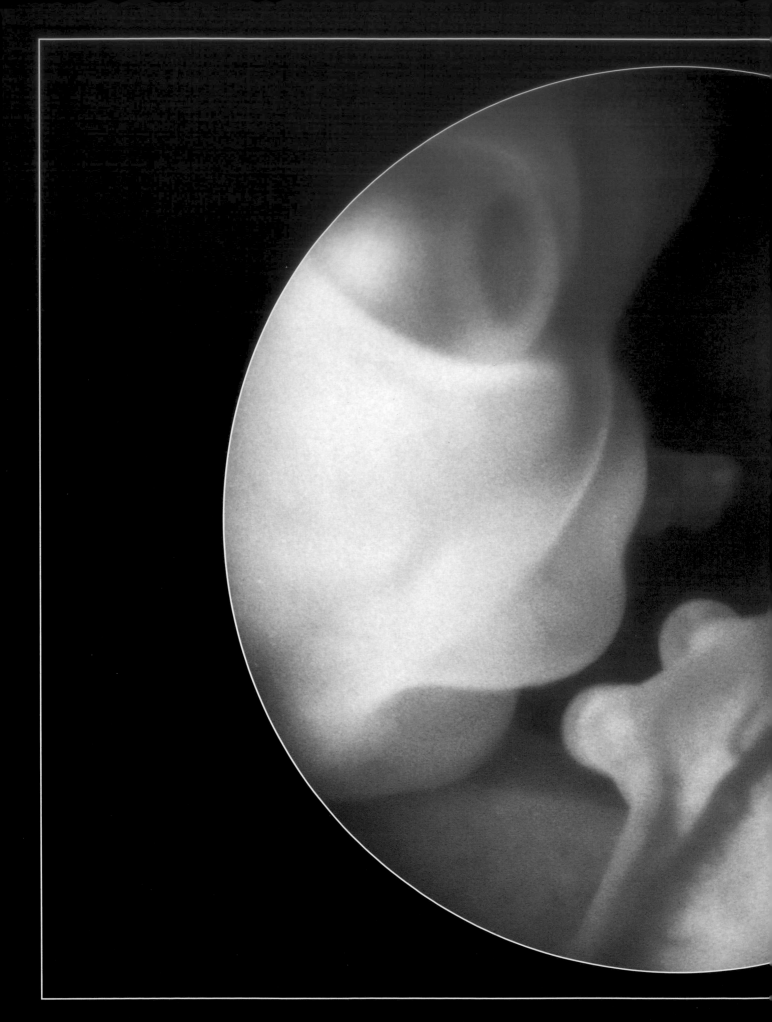

Profile
in the stunning distortion of a
wide-angle lens. In the background
is the embryo's rich-red placenta.

about eighty times a minute. As before, these functions are not mere rehearsals; they keep the embryo alive from day to day.

The embryo begins to look obviously alive when it starts to move. The first intimation of activity is an occasional ripple going through the whole body and a barely perceptible sideward wiggle when the embryo is about five weeks old, probably as soon as nerve channels and muscles link up.

The repertoire becomes more varied during the next two weeks. The embryo slowly and gracefully begins to bend and extend its arms and legs, turns its head from side to side, swings the whole body to and fro, and sometimes stretches from head to toe. Occasionally there is a sudden jerky startle with arms and legs flung out, looking like the startles of newborn babies.

The movements are not only for practice. They are considered vital for the healthy development of muscles and joints. But while the embryo is still so small the mother cannot perceive any of these activities, which have become known in such detail only since the advent of ultrasound monitoring. The development of movement has been found to be as orderly as the building of the body. Like the body's structural development, prenatal movements unfold in a definite sequence and each movement has a defined form. The sequence and the form of movements are inherent and derived from the same genetic program that governed the molding of the body. Movements have

Hand paddles show the beginnings for fingers, at the outset of this month.

recognizable shape, just as the body does. Thus, even in the blur of an ultrasound image, it is possible to learn to recognize "this is an arm" and "this is an arm waving up and down."

Seeing a movement depends on catching the embryo in the act. Unlike physical development, movements are fleeting events. Therefore the diary for the onset of each new activity is known only by approximate age in weeks, not to the day. It may be that the time schedule in the development of behavior is not quite as regimented as the physical development of the body has been and continues to be in this month.

According to the daily diary of physical development, we know that the embryo's brain makes a quick advance at the beginning

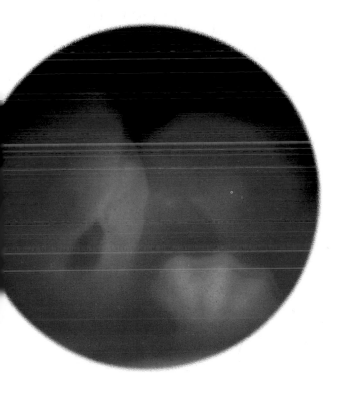

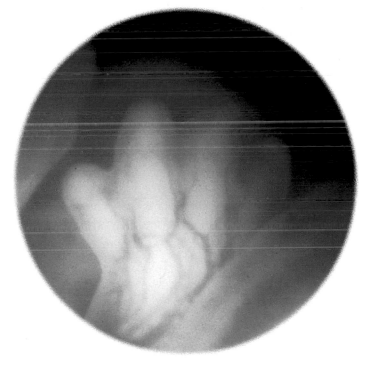

Finger ridges
increase daily; the arms do not yet reach across the red bulge of the beating heart.

Fingers and thumb
have emerged at six weeks, when the embryo starts to wiggle and will soon move its arms.

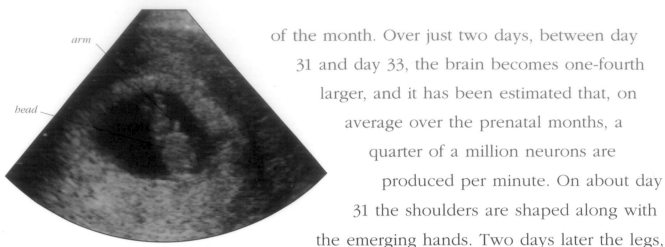

arm

head

An arm waving can be recognized in the blur of an ultrasound image in the seventh week.

of the month. Over just two days, between day 31 and day 33, the brain becomes one-fourth larger, and it has been estimated that, on average over the prenatal months, a quarter of a million neurons are produced per minute. On about day 31 the shoulders are shaped along with the emerging hands. Two days later the legs, always lagging behind the arms until the second year of life, begin to show prospective thigh, calf, and foot regions, while the hand paddles already have distinct ridges for fingers and thumbs. At the same time, the retina of the eyes gains pigment. The far from finished eyes are always open; their lids will form at the end of this month. On about day 33, the nostril openings develop elevated rims which go into building the nose. Four days later, on about day 37, the tip of the nose first shows up in profile and is formed with nostrils and the two separate air passages, anticipating the arrival of air in the future.

While the rapid body building is in progress the teeming cell activity continues. Throughout this time the highly active cells are particularly vulnerable. Some of the mother's activities affect the life within her. We do not know the many subtle ways in which this may occur. We do know some of the simple facts of the embryo's participation in the mother's nutrition, in what she drinks, in the cigarette smoke she may inhale. Alcohol quickly reaches the embryo, and in the same concentration as in the mother's blood. Nicotine and carbon monoxide (both present in cigarette smoke), caffeine, most drugs and gases, virus infections – all can get through. It is sometimes suggested that the tendency for mothers to feel tired and not adventurous during these early weeks, to dislike certain foods, or have food fads, may all have a natural protective effect for the embryo.

By midmonth, the embryo has moved ahead. Details are filled in. The mouth has lips and the beginnings of a tongue, there is a good upper and lower jaw, and the buds for all twenty milk teeth are in the gums. Tear ducts are forming in the eyes. The two ears have developed in unison and have taken shape according to the family pattern; some embryos have larger ears than others, some have prominent ear lobes, others almost no lobes. The fingers have grown longer, and by the end of the month will bear the fine ridges of fingerprints, hallmarks of this child's unique individuality.

Tip of the nose shows up in profile. With arms grown longer the embryo can reach up to it.

While these details are developing, the whole embryo is moving toward an increase in size and weight. The umbilical cord becomes large enough to carry increasing nourishment for future growth. The completed skeleton begins to harden with its many complex links and joints. The first bone-marrow cells appear on about day 49. This day has been given special significance.

Day 49 has been elected to be the final day of the scientifically recorded day-to-day diary of development. On this day, the embryo is seven weeks old and is considered to be essentially complete. The creative enterprise of prolific cell division, differentiation, streaming migrations, establishment of new cell communities, and specialization: these come to rest when

▷ *A bold hand*
confronts the
camera. The fingers
have prominent
touch pads; the
cord is alongside.

the foundations for all the working parts of the body are in place. From now on increasing individual differences in timing assert themselves and the development of the body is no longer known to the day. All development in body and behavior henceforth will be counted in weeks, not days.

The embryo outgrows its name and from here on is called a *fetus*, from the Latin word meaning "offspring" or "young one." In the next month the young one will plainly show its sex externally. Since the baby to be born at the end of this book is a girl, the pronoun used here will be "she" although everything said is equally true for a boy.

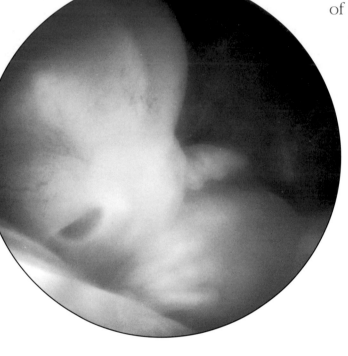

A new name
at the end of the month
the embryo becomes a
fetus, here nestling
against the folds of its
amnion membrane.

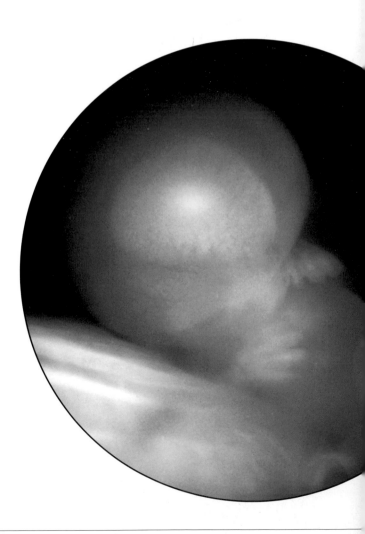

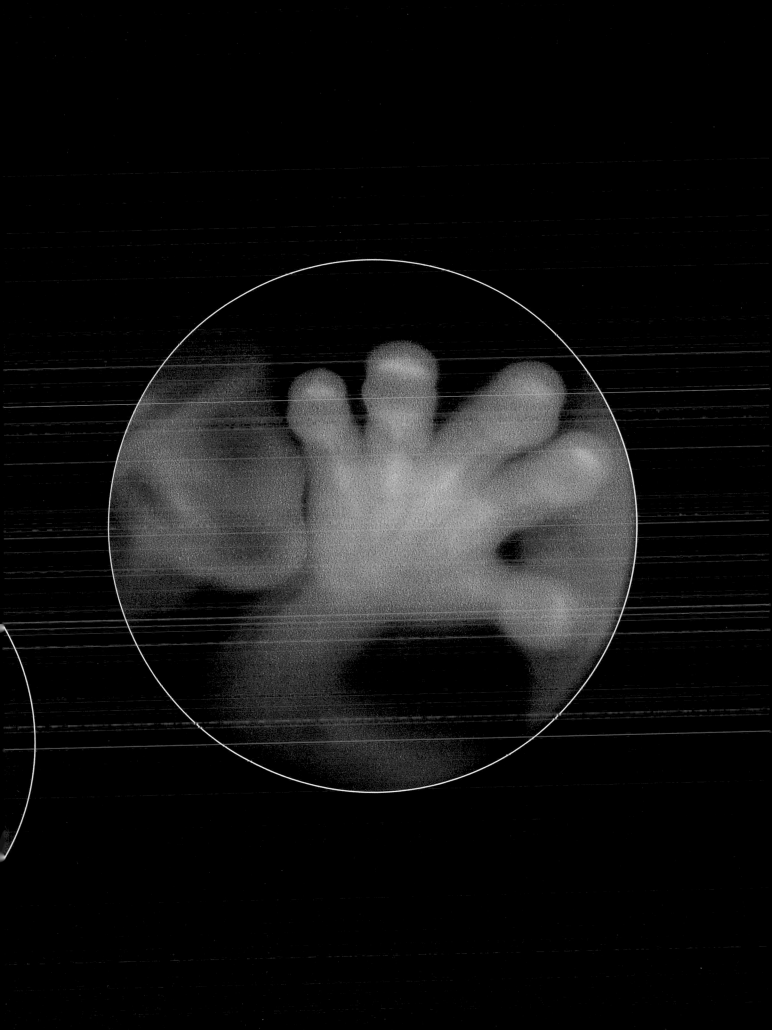

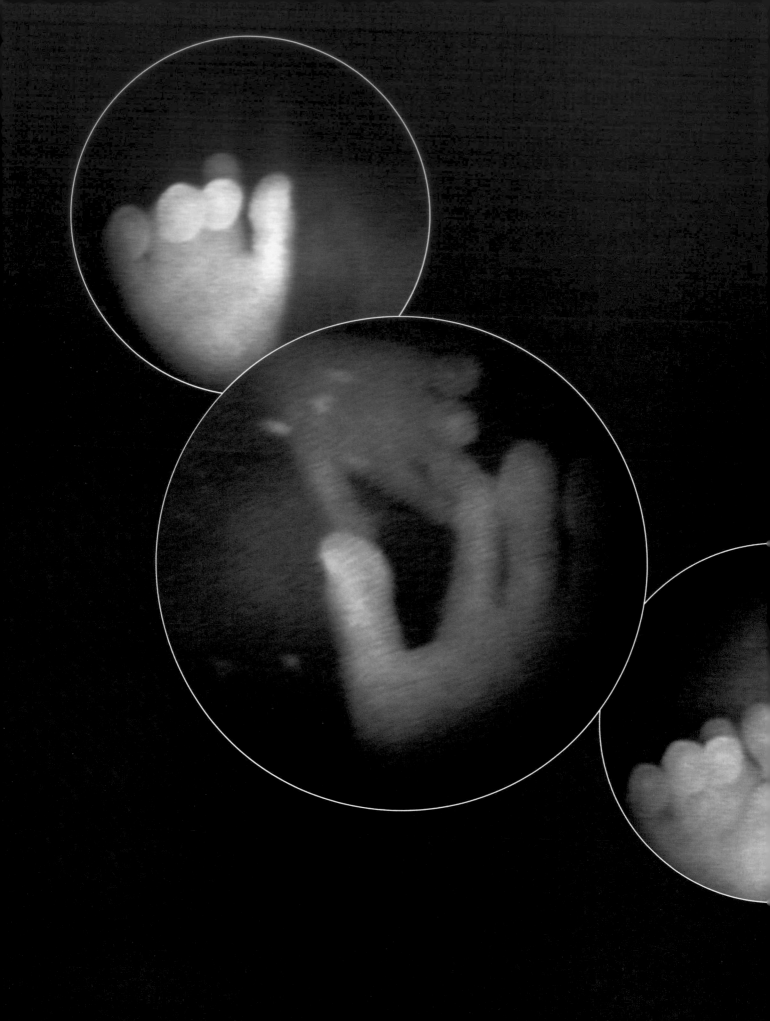

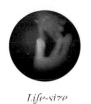

Life-size

The baby becomes very lively this month. In the freedom of the watery pool the tiny being moves gracefully and with ease and progresses to outdo any newborn in acrobatic feats.

The third month

Collision of erratic spores
Moved eyes to bud, fingers to swell
Out of the light, and now he walks
On water, and is miracle.
ANTHONY THWAITE: *To My Unborn Child*

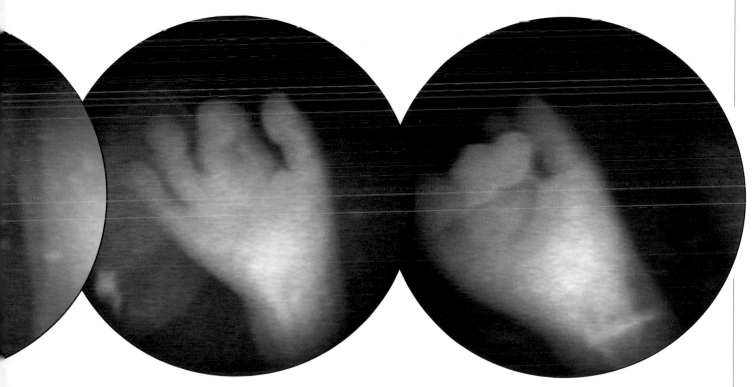

Graceful hands, fingers opening and closing, from a video sequence.

The baby can now roll over from front to back and elegantly all around and from time to time smoothly launches into somersaults, backward and forward. In more modest activities she sways from side to side, makes leisurely stepping movements, and expansively opens her arms wide. Occasionally she may have a full-length stretch, sometimes accompanied by a wide yawn or, as if breathing out, seemingly heaves a deep sigh. As in breathing, the baby's chest and abdomen make brief respiratory excursions now and then. She frequently has bouts of hiccups, sometimes has sudden startles, and often touches her own face which is especially sensitive around the mouth. She almost certainly sucks her thumb or fingers; she regularly drinks down sips of amniotic fluid, and urinates into her pool which is freshened in a continual turnover of fluids.

In this month she not only begins to behave like a newborn she also, in miniature proportions, looks more like a newborn, albeit a very skinny newborn reaching over some three inches in sitting height. Although she gains about tenfold from last month's peanut-weight, this amounts to hardly more than an ounce. She is still too small and feeble for the mother to feel the cavorting going on within. Yet the baby actually reaches a peak frequency of movement in the secrecy of her seclusion. In a wide variety of quick and slow, small and large movements, she rarely pauses for more than five minutes and does not yet have any sleep; that will come only with greater maturity. She is vertical as often as horizontal and may change her position perhaps twenty times an hour even while the mother is lying quite still. The legendary curled-up fetal position exists only in our imagination: the baby does not seem to know of it.

The baby's back is beautifully mobile. It may be straight and upright one minute and gracefully arched backward the next, with the head tilted back. Then again, she may bend forward and bring her head to the chest and can turn her head fully right and left even in that position. Her legs and arms may be folded one moment and extended the next. She can move so fluently because she is afloat, not quite weightless but under reduced gravity, and she is still small enough to have plenty of elbow room.

On top of the baby's own activities she is also affected like a boat at sea by the mother's movements. Every time the mother takes a breath, the baby is slightly rocked. When the mother coughs, when she laughs, when she walks, there is a commotion in the baby's pool of fluids and the baby is swayed back and forth. The effect of a mother lightly dancing is different from a mother striding down the street. Not only are the mother's movements transmitted but the sound of heels on pavement, the sound of voices, and all louder noises also come through. It is not known how early sound might be experienced by the baby. We do know that the inner hearing apparatus is formed, although not yet mature in this month, and there is some research evidence that the baby might show some sensitivity to sound by the twelfth week. Certainly, sounds will become a major part of the baby's life in the coming months.

Small feet float into view against the marbled background of the womb.

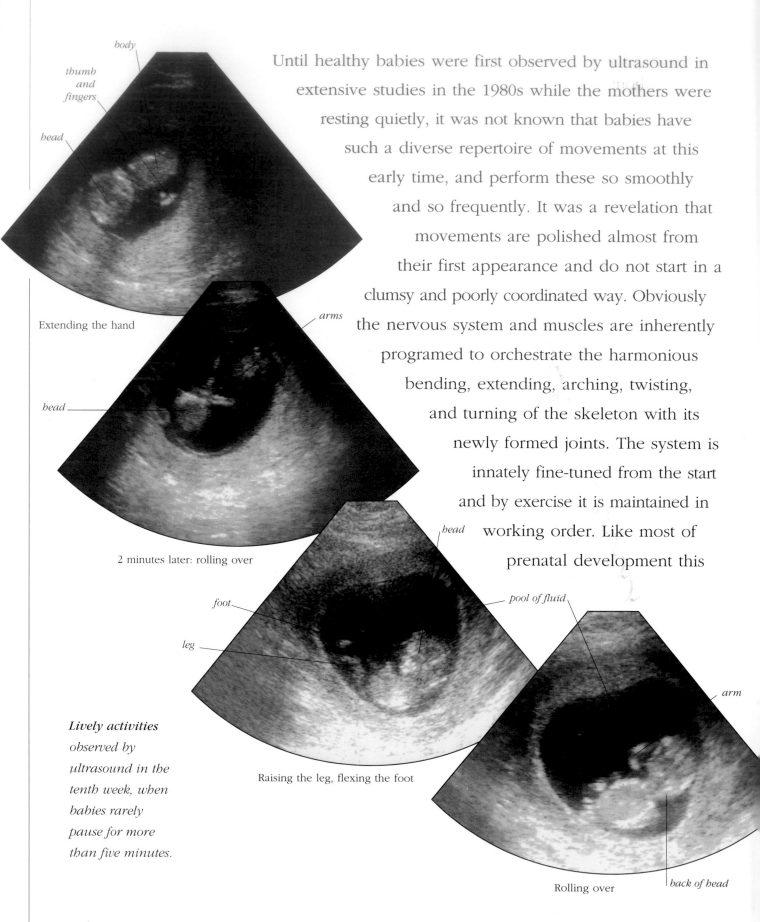

body

thumb
and
fingers

head

Extending the hand

head

2 minutes later: rolling over

Lively activities
observed by
ultrasound in the
tenth week, when
babies rarely
pause for more
than five minutes.

arms

foot

leg

Raising the leg, flexing the foot

head

pool of fluid

arm

back of head

Rolling over

Until healthy babies were first observed by ultrasound in extensive studies in the 1980s while the mothers were resting quietly, it was not known that babies have such a diverse repertoire of movements at this early time, and perform these so smoothly and so frequently. It was a revelation that movements are polished almost from their first appearance and do not start in a clumsy and poorly coordinated way. Obviously the nervous system and muscles are inherently programed to orchestrate the harmonious bending, extending, arching, twisting, and turning of the skeleton with its newly formed joints. The system is innately fine-tuned from the start and by exercise it is maintained in working order. Like most of prenatal development this both caters for today and anticipates tomorrow. It is "anticipatory development" toward what will become essential at birth.

Being able to breathe will be a top priority at birth. For such a vital function it is not surprising that there is a lot of advance preparation and practice. In addition to having good lungs, there is also the need for the body to be ready to draw breath and expel it, similar to the function of bellows. That is the job of the diaphragm, working in conjunction with the rib cage and abdomen. The diaphragm begins to work in this month. It starts up in short sessions, repeated a few times an hour, expanding and contracting as it will eventually do full-time after birth. Here, instead of air, small amounts of amniotic fluid wash in and out. The fluid is not harmful, on the contrary it is thought to aid the development of the lung tissues. The diaphragm gets further exercise through hiccuping. As many as one hundred hiccups an hour have been counted in babies in these early months. The hiccups come in repeated bouts lasting several minutes, then stop, and start all over again. They have been recognized as a scientific puzzle for nearly a hundred years; the best guess is that these prenatal hiccups may be important for the strengthening of the diaphragm and the working of the whole respiratory apparatus. When we hiccup in later life, this harks back to our earliest time.

face

legs

Sliding up

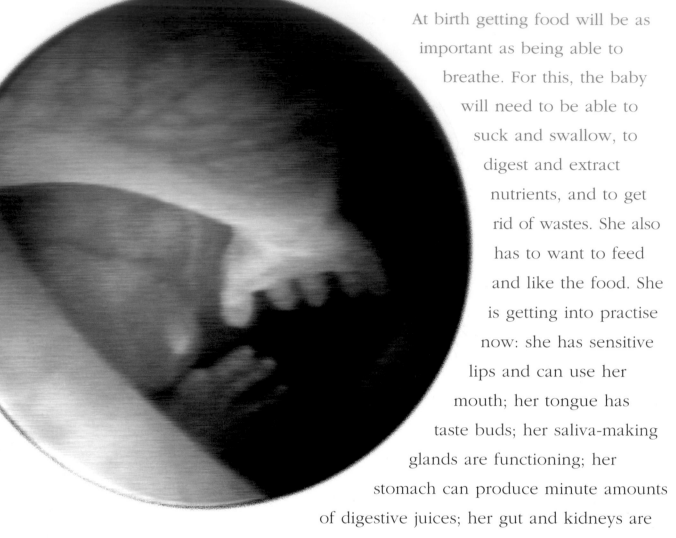

She moves smoothly and has bouts of hiccups, drinks and urinates, and practises her breathing.

At birth getting food will be as important as being able to breathe. For this, the baby will need to be able to suck and swallow, to digest and extract nutrients, and to get rid of wastes. She also has to want to feed and like the food. She is getting into practise now: she has sensitive lips and can use her mouth; her tongue has taste buds; her saliva-making glands are functioning; her stomach can produce minute amounts of digestive juices; her gut and kidneys are working. When she takes in sips of amniotic fluid and swallows it, her digestive system can process it. Some nutrients are extracted, mainly sugars and salts, and a small amount of solid waste accumulates. It will remain stored in her intestine, while fluid waste is continually carried out in driblets of urine. The urine is sterile and does not foul the amniotic waters.

By the end of this month one can tell boy from girl at a glance. Each shows distinctly male or female genitalia. Penis and vulva have become formed out of foundations which looked superficially unisex at the beginning of this month, when prospective clitoris and penis still had very similar shape and size. The baby's internal reproductive organs have long been active, and it is their output of male or female hormones which have created the outward sexual distinctions. But even by the end of this month, a boy's testicles have not descended and will not move into the scrotum until shortly before birth, sometimes even later. A girl's ovaries inside her body now already contain a store of primitive ova, and by the time of birth will hold, in unripened form, all the eggs she will ever possess.

There are striking external changes in this month. The overall proportions change: the growth of the head slows down and the rest of the body catches up; the neck is formed; the arms and legs grow to look long; the fingers too grow longer and more tapering, and fingernails grow. The baby's face begins to show its individual features, probably bearing family resemblances. Not only the shape of the ears, but also the shape of the eyes and of the whole face are now distinctive for each baby.

During this time, usually in the ninth or tenth week, the eyelids grow large enough to cover the eyes. As soon as they do, the baby's eyes close, and stay closed. Upper and lower lids become sealed and will not open again for the next three months. By then the baby will be much larger and much more solid. She will make impressive progress toward this in the next month.

Closed eyes stay sealed for three months. Their blue color, the same in all prenatal babies, shimmers through the delicate lids

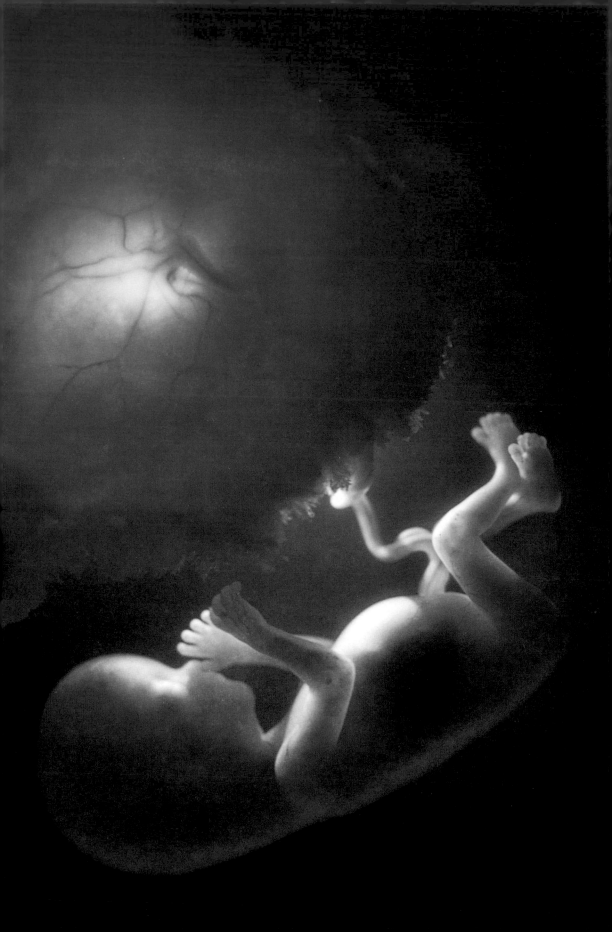

Growing three inches in four weeks,
the baby becomes about eight inches tall
from head to toe. She increases her
weight sevenfold but even so comes to
weigh only about seven ounces.

The fourth month

Her vital organs round out her belly,
her limbs are lean and lanky, she has
no fat, and her skin is so transparent
that it reveals the fine tracery of the
underlying blood vessels.

Life-size
the slim-limbed
baby and the great
placenta, near the
end of this month.

In this month the baby becomes big and strong enough finally to assert her active presence as her mother can begin to feel the impact of the stirring, quickening life within. This may start around the sixteenth week, sometimes earlier, sometimes later. At first the baby's long-practiced movements may seem like vague internal flutterings, as by a butterfly. After some days the sensation becomes unmistakable evidence of the baby's lively activities: turning, kicking, somersaulting as before, albeit now with less free space.

For her prodigious growth the baby needs increasingly greater quantities of sustenance to provide both substance and energy. The resources come from the mother and are made available to the baby through the actions of the baby's own placenta, which becomes fully established this month. The placenta is named after the Latin word for cake. It looks more like a cushion and it is a lot more than cake. It does not deserve to be dismissed as the mere afterbirth, for it is an admirably versatile organ and an essential part of the developing baby. It plays the star role in the support system that began its specialized development among the cells of the early cluster.

It is the evolution of the placenta that makes pregnancy possible. Thanks to the placenta, a baby can grow within the great protection of a mother's body, much safer than any egg in a nest. And the arrangement gives a mother freedom to move about in a relatively unhampered way, not tied down like a hen sitting to hatch her brood.

The placenta "cushion" contains a soft structure of blood vessels belonging to the baby and branching out to look like a tree, a tree of life. The branching placental vessels incorporate the earlier rootlike villi and are surrounded by maternal blood, carrying nutrients, vitamins, minerals, water, oxygen, and all the good substances the mother has available. But the mother's blood never enters the baby's vessels. Instead, invisibly small molecules of the supplies traverse the porous vessel walls of the placental tree and so enter the baby's bloodstream.

The placenta is not merely a transfer depot. It appears to have the capacity to actively select, process, and regulate what and how much is taken in, according to the baby's changing needs. The placenta is also thought to have some protective functions. It is described as being like a sponge that can soak up and perhaps neutralize some harmful agents that may arrive, especially agents of infections. Unfortunately the protection is not perfect. As the embryologist George Corner wrote: "By accepting the shelter of the uterus the fetus also takes the risk of maternal disease or malnutrition...." As before, substances like alcohol, caffeine, or the products of cigarette smoke do go in also.

At the same time there is an outgoing traffic in which the placenta facilitates waste disposal. There is a constant departure of wastes, again in the form of molecules, traveling out from the baby's bloodstream through the placental vessel walls, to be washed away in the mother's circulation. The placental vessels can cater to the growing demands of the baby because these branching vessels become so profuse by the time of birth that, if spread out flat, their total surface would cover more than half a tennis court!

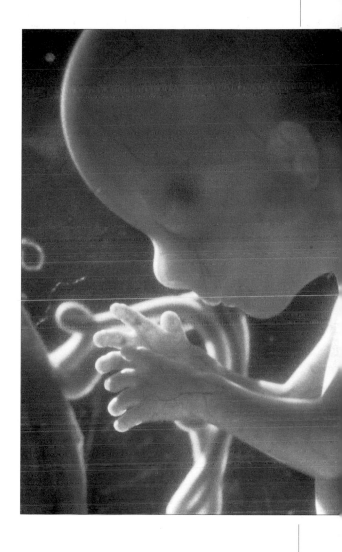

Face and hands become more shapely, the body is more substantial; here one-and-a-half times life-size.

▷ *Tree of life*
the placenta's
branching
vessels laid bare.

The remarkable placenta may be called a guardian of the pregnancy. In its panoply of functions it also has vital effects on the mother's body to make a successful pregnancy possible. In the fourth month the placenta takes over the production of the hormone *progesterone*, meaning "for pregnancy." This is the key hormone that stimulates the mother's body, particularly her uterus, toward continuing physical hospitality to the baby. The baby is thereby endowed with the biological means to evoke the prenatal conditions it needs. Not only this, but far ahead of birth, progesterone also interacts with a team of hormones acting on the mother's breasts to make them ready for producing milk. At the same time the hormonal team boosts the efficiency of the mother's metabolism so that her body can more easily provide for two, and it usually promotes the pregnant mother's good health and sense of well-being. If she has suffered from morning sickness, it will tend to pass this month. Thus the placenta fosters the baby's interest in being carried by a mother who is healthy and feels well.

The living cord
plugs into the
placenta "cushion."

In its guardianlike functions the placenta makes still further contributions. It produces heat that tops up the mother's body temperature and maintains the baby about one degree warmer than the mother. Later, in the last three months of pregnancy, it will enter into the transfer from mother to baby of vital factors for immunities against infections. Finally, the placenta will play an important role in setting the time for birth and will then end its useful life along with the umbilical cord.

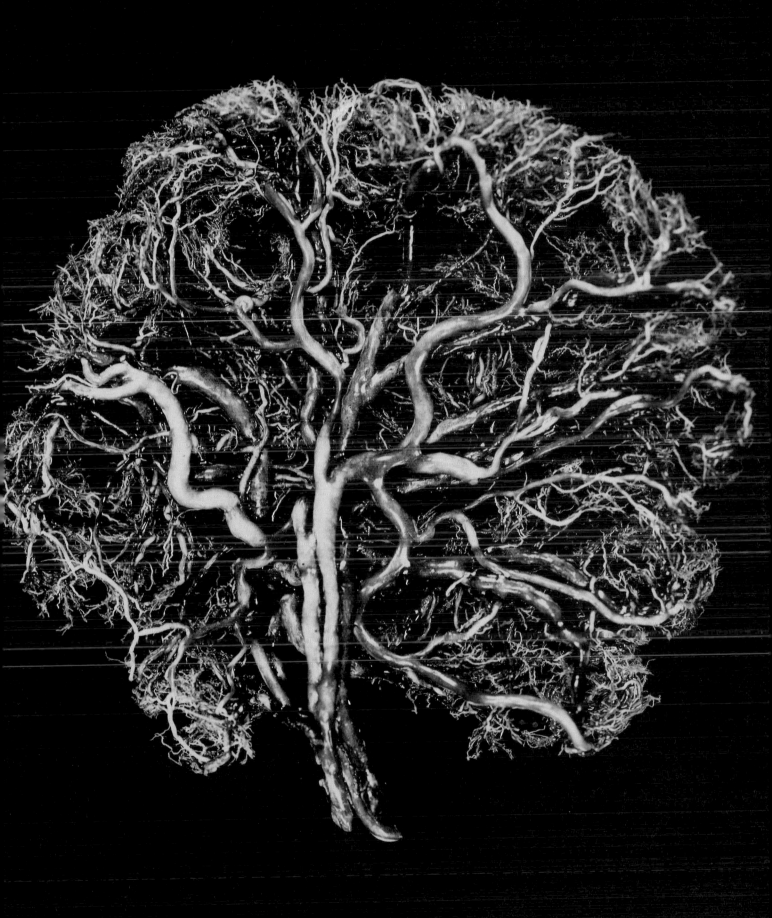

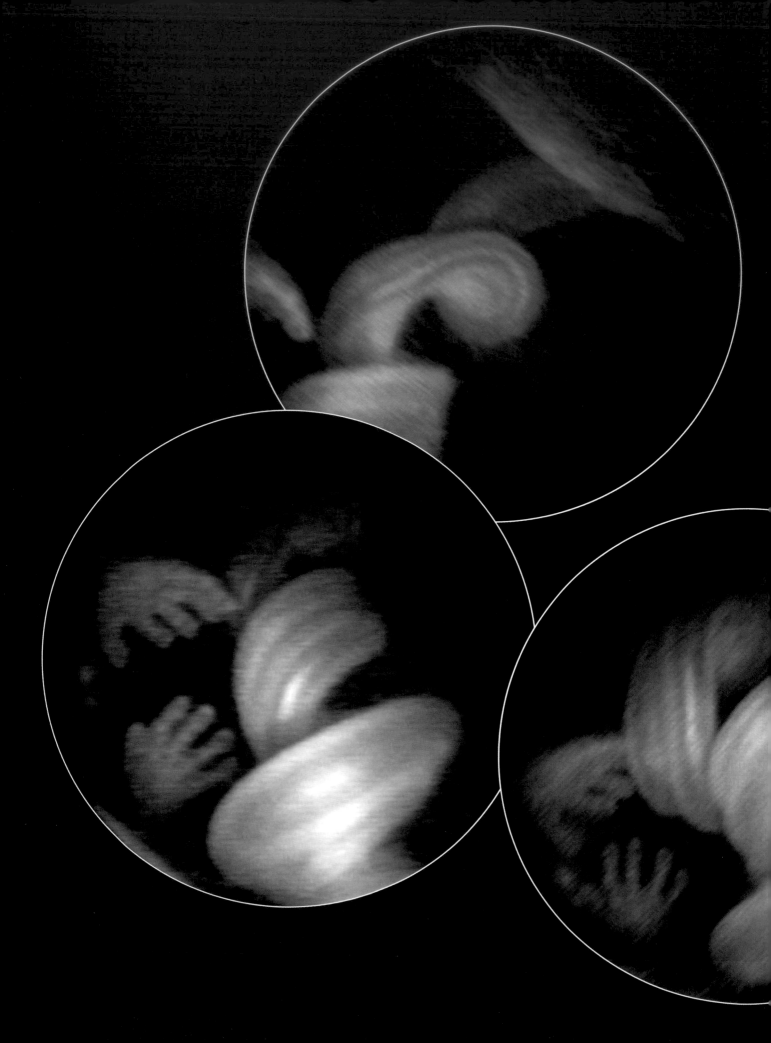

The umbilical cord, so often celebrated as the link between mother and child, is actually the link between the baby and its own placenta and no less remarkable for that. At four months the cord can carry a circulation equivalent to twenty-five quarts a day; by the time of birth it will carry three hundred quarts a day. This circulation flows in constant round trips, bringing supplies to the baby from the placental tree, and returning wastes to the placenta, so swiftly that a round trip is completed in about thirty seconds. The throbbing circulation is pumped entirely by the baby's heart; only the baby's own blood, never the mother's, enters into it.

The cord is continually distended by the baby's bloodstream and therefore, like a water-filled garden hose, it resists knotting and tends to straighten out if tangled as the baby moves about. As a symbol of health and life it is thought that the cord was adopted by surgeon-barbers in the past for the design of the traditional spiraling, red and white barber's pole. Although the cord is not rigid, it too is spiraling, has a pale white color and its three colorfully red and twisting vessels shimmer through the surface.

In the womb the baby depends on the cord as a deep-sea diver or a space-walking astronaut does on a lifeline. The system allows the baby to live underwater within its sealed sac, the "bag of waters." The sac is a strong and slightly stretchy transparent membrane. It is called *amnion* from the Greek word for "little lamb," a name given because lambs are often born enclosed in this membrane. Human babies may also be born with some of their

Spiraling lifeline
the pulsating cord
is within reach of
the baby's hands in
the womb.

amnion draped over the head, born "under a caul" which, in folklore, is deemed to be an omen for good fortune. The amnion membrane is made entirely of living cells descended from the original cell cluster. The amnion grows larger along with the baby. It provides housing and its cells also produce some of the fluid, the amniotic fluid, which makes up the "waters" for the baby. The rest of the fluid is produced by the baby's own lungs and kidneys, and some fluid components may seep in from the surrounding uterus.

Until this month the very small baby was afloat in only a small amount of amniotic fluid. In the fourth month this quantity greatly increases to about one quart. It is still unknown what sets off and what controls this month's influx, fulfilling the requirements for the bigger baby to be comfortably afloat. Only when the volume of liquid has increased does it become possible to withdraw the considerable amount of this fluid required for the medical test of *amniocentesis*, which means "amnion puncture" – an experience for the baby that may be similar to pulling a bath plug, and babies do respond with some signs of agitation, sometimes for many hours afterward. The amnion quickly reseals itself, and in time the quantity of fluid builds up again under the intriguing internal regulation that keeps the pool well filled.

When babies were observed by monitoring during this month it was found that the frequency of each baby's activity was much the same morning, noon, and evening, with no distinctions as yet across the day. This will come next month. But there are activity differences between one baby and another; some are consistently more active, and others more sedate, as their mothers will probably notice in the coming months. Active or sedate, each baby's bouts of activity begin to last minutes longer, and pauses also stretch, but the baby still does not sleep and rarely rests for more than six or seven minutes. The mother cannot feel every movement. She can feel only the larger ones and only those that happen to touch upon her sensitive nerve endings, mainly the movements directed outward toward her abdominal wall.

There are many subtle activities that a mother can never feel. She cannot feel the baby delicately moving fingers and wiggling toes, or performing a pincer grip with thumb and fingers, or making a fist, or the exercise of breathing, all of which are counted in recording the constant round of activities. We know that in this month the baby gradually steps up her breathing practice, doing this more often and in slightly longer sessions. Then, toward the end of the month the baby adds another very subtle activity. She begins to make excursions with her eyes beneath her fused lids. At first she scans only from one side to the other, to the right and the left. In the next months she will do much more of this, and her activities and responses to her environment will become more clear and obvious.

The throbbing cord is a constant presence in the baby's round of activities.

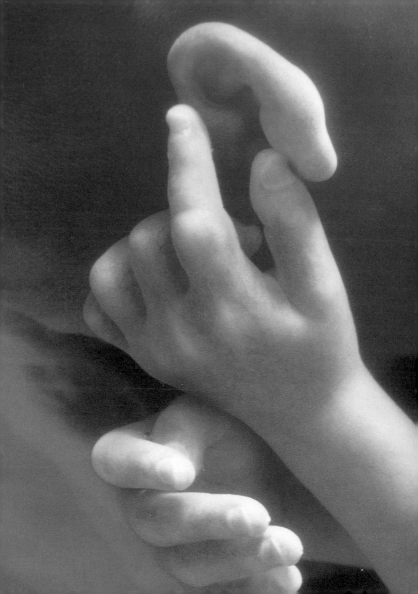

If the mother becomes attuned she may – as ancient biblical wisdom proclaimed – learn to recognize in these two months how her baby

The fifth and sixth months

For lo, as soon as the voice of thy salutation sounded in my ears, the babe in my womb leapt for joy. St. Luke 1:44

Sound is heard *voices, music, loud noises, all these reach the baby.*

responds to the world around: to voices and especially her own voice, to music, to sudden noises, to a pat on her abdomen, and also to her own emotions, be they pleasure, excitement, anxiety, or fear.

As the baby grows to be bigger and heftier, as her hearing and nervous system become more mature, her activities and responses become more obvious. By the end of the fifth month she is likely to weigh one pound and be ten or more inches tall, surpassing half her expected length at birth. In the sixth month she may go on to grow two more inches and gain close to another pound. She will definitely be noticed now. Not only by the mother, but also by those allowed to put a hand on the mother's abdomen to feel the movements. Even the world at large can plainly see the bulge of a baby on the way.

Hand on amnion touching the fine folds of membrane (photographed in an earlier month.)

The baby still has just enough room to move fairly freely and be comfortably afloat. A good deal is known of her likely activities. At any one moment she might be sitting upright, with straightened back and legs crossed in a yogalike position, or she could be lounging as if she were in a hammock with her arms folded under her head, or more energetically she may pedal her legs, make crawling movements, roll over, or turn somersaults. In the sixth month the balance organs in her inner ears become mature and so she may be able to choose and maintain her own position. Much of the time she may choose to be head-down, perhaps because blood rushing to her head may be a comfortable sensation in the normally low-oxygen conditions in the womb. Tens of thousands of babies have been monitored and from these observations a picture can be pieced together of how babies generally spend their days and learn about their surroundings.

The pulsating, throbbing umbilical cord is the baby's constant companion and babies reach toward it, touch it, bump into it, move around it, and hear its rushing stream of circulation. The amnion membrane too is always within reach and babies can be seen snuggling their faces against it, or slowly running their hand over the folds of the amnion surface as if to explore it. With their excellent sense of touch, one of the earliest senses to become mature, it is not surprising that babies are also seen touching and stroking their own bodies and becoming well acquainted with themselves. They particularly seem to like to touch their own face over and over again, sometimes bringing the hands to the face, and sometimes leaning far forward to bring face to hands. A majority of babies show a preference for the right hand over the left, and this may reinforce brain development in this direction. Right- or left-handed, babies can by now adeptly manipulate their fingers, move the thumb in opposition to the fingers, or make a fist. They are often seen sucking their thumb or fingers, and most of them can find their mouth more readily than they will be able to do when born. Gravity will then hinder them, and the sight of their own hands may distract their sense of touch practiced in darkness.

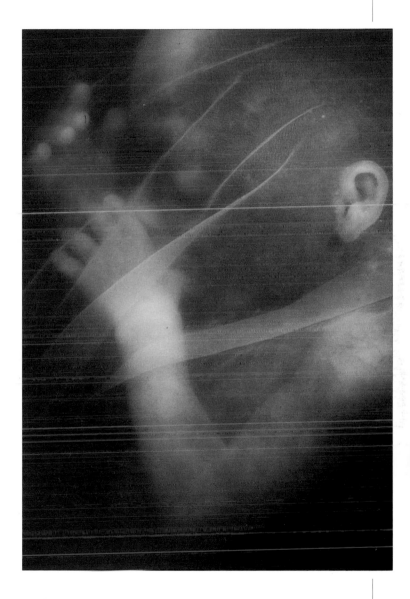

Inside the amnion at 19 weeks there is just enough room to sit upright and move fairly freely.

The activities often look playful. A researcher one day observed identical-twin boys, residing in a shared amnion sac, having a "boxing match with repeated rounds of a few minutes each," as one twin batted his brother and the other patted back. After resting for a few minutes, they started another round. Another pair of twin brothers, separated in adjacent amnion sacs, engaged each other in a similar exchange, landing their gentle blows by pushing against the flexible amnion membranes that divided them. Convivial experience starts early, no doubt for girl twins as well as boys.

It is not all fun and games. Babies do also experience and show the effects of stress. Following an earthquake in Italy in 1980, twenty-eight pregnant mothers who had been badly frightened but

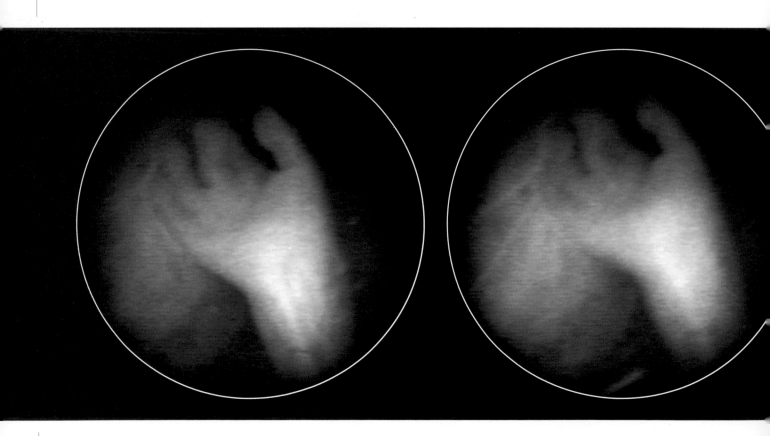

Reaching up to the amnion
the baby's hand in the light-refracting fluids

...a split second later
in this video sequence, the hand has advanced

not injured were observed under ultrasound. All of the twenty-eight babies in the womb were found to be intensely overactive, and the hyperactivity lasted for several hours after the earthquake. Some of these babies then slowed down to normal liveliness. But the rest fell into abnormal inactivity for as long as three days before they perked up again. The alarm that the mothers experienced appeared to have been in some way transmitted to their babies.

Ordinary everyday stresses may also stir the baby. For instance, if the mother is very tired but keeps going, or if she is upset, the baby tends to move more. Although there are no nerve channels, nor any other direct physical connections between mother and child, adrenaline and other arousing or depressant substances can

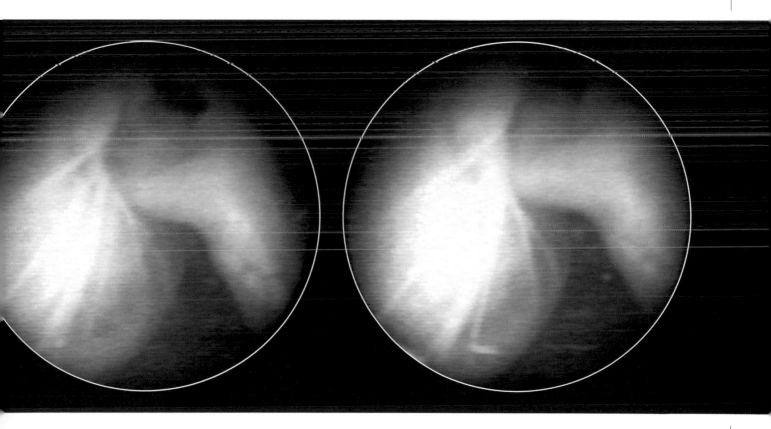

... another split second later
the fingers sink into the membrane folds

... and all the way into the amnion
showing how twins might bat each other.

cross the placenta and affect the baby. Other aspects of maternal stress might be transmitted through the mother's more agitated movements, through her general muscle tension, the tone and loudness of her voice, or changes in her heartbeat. The shelter of the womb is not a soundproof chamber, nor is it isolated from the wider world the mother lives in.

Noise certainly travels through from outside. Although the hearing apparatus will not be fully mature until about the twenty-eighth week, babies begin to show some auditory responses after the sixteenth week, possibly even earlier. Cars honking, bells ringing, doors slamming, washing machines whizzing, jet engines screeching, people shouting, music crescendos, audiences

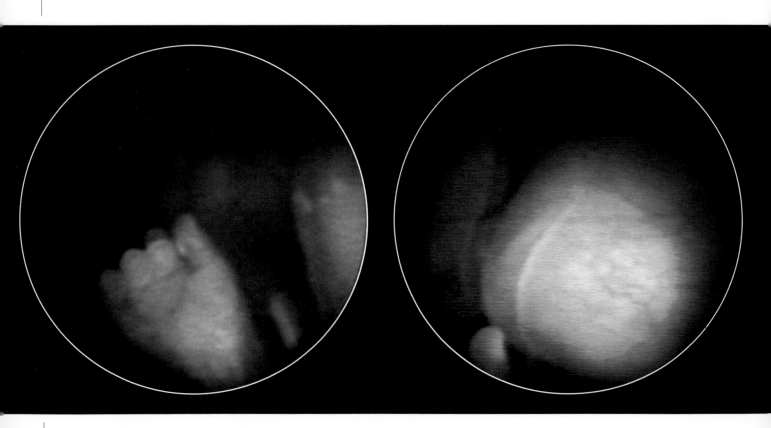

Snuggling into the amnion: the head is at center, hand and shoulder in the foreground

... the face rolls over the amnion, with thumb near the mouth, seen from below the chin, in a video sequence in the fourth month.

applauding – all these make an impact and stir babies into activity, as many mothers notice. Pleasant or unpleasant, the baby is already living among the sounds of the outside world she will inhabit. For better or worse she may become accustomed to certain noises. In one study it was found that newborn babies, whose mothers lived near a noisy airport during pregnancy, were likely to sleep through the noise of landing jet planes that would awaken other newborns. As more scientific knowledge is gathered about prenatal hearing, one cannot quite dismiss old folklore as expressed in a colorful West African saying:

> "A man should never get angry at his wife while she is
> pregnant, for his raised voice turns seven times in her
> vagina and reaches the child to be."

A pleasant way for parents to spend time with their baby may be to play prenatal games. In programs that have been called "hothousing" it is suggested that parents could begin touch-dialogues with the baby in these weeks. Although there is no good scientific evidence for claims that the baby's intelligence might be enhanced by this, it can be entertaining for parents, quite likely also for the baby, and a good way to be literally in touch and cultivate the relationship. To play the game it is suggested that the parents wait for a movement from the baby and then reply with a gentle pat to that location on the abdomen. The baby may respond with a nudge from inside. Parents have reported that over the next months this can be expanded to an exchange of multiple tapping back and forth. When the parents discover where the baby's head, bottom, hands and feet are, they may enjoy the game even more.

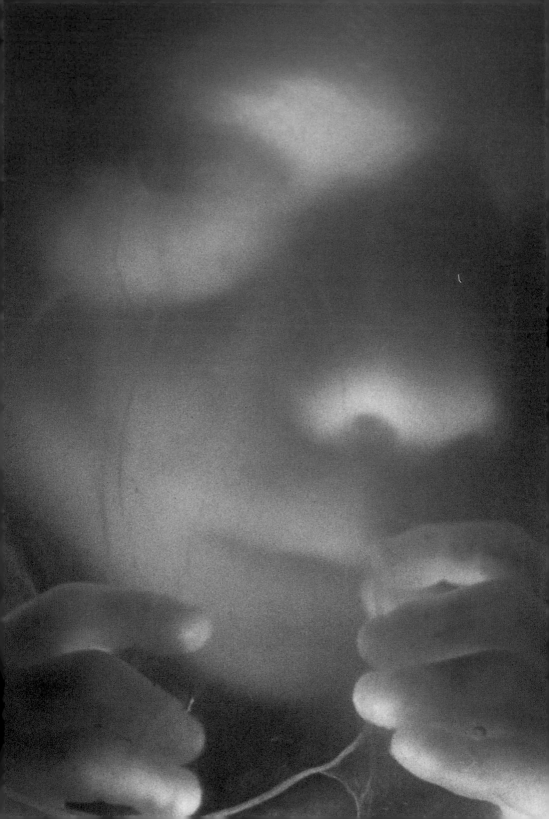

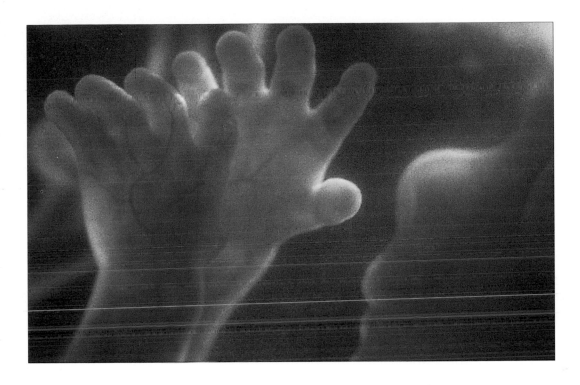

In the fifth month (at left) and the sixth (opposite) the fingers can play delicately, the closed eyes can dart back and forth.

In privacy the baby goes on further developing the many quiet activities that cannot be felt. With sophisticated monitoring techniques it is possible to discern fine details of eye movements, even while the eyelids are still sealed shut. In these two months the baby improves her ability to move her eyes. When she started to do this last month, she occasionally swept her eyes from side to side but only with her eyes cast downward. By her twentieth week, she can lift her eyes level and turn them slowly from side to side, on and on, for prolonged periods. At other times her eyes dart quickly back and forth, sometimes smoothly, sometimes jerkily. The two eyes do not always move in tandem. One eye may veer off, or the eyes may turn in opposite directions to be momentarily cross-eyed or wall-eyed; fine-tuned coordination will not come until some time after birth. After one or two weeks of only horizontal eye movements, the baby starts to be able to roll her eyes up and down, and all around.

The baby finally opens her eyes near the end of the sixth month when the eyelids become unsealed. She scans the darkness and can now open and close her eyes. She may blink if there is a sudden noise and thereby establishes that she has heard. Although the visual system is not yet mature she has some experience of dimly diffused light, especially if the mother is standing in bright light. The darkness of the womb is not pitch-black and the baby may sense the difference between bright sunlight and the darkness of night.

A profile portrait at 20 weeks by ultrasound. She has billions of neurons in her maturing brain.

Quietly, the baby goes on making breathing movements, more often and for longer periods than before and more often at night than in the day. From the twentieth week onward, slight but detectable and regular differences begin to appear in activity levels between morning, noon, and night, and these differences will become much more pronounced in the coming months. Morning tends to be the quietest time; the busiest is toward midnight, as many a mother discovers. The emergence of daily cycles of activity is a sign of increasing maturity. At about twenty weeks, the baby has virtually all the neurons she will ever have in her brain, billions of neurons. This is also the time when she begins to show variations in the rate of her heartbeat. When the heart rate changes become more marked next month, they can be used to measure the baby's responses to various events, especially to sounds and noises that may make her heart beat faster. She may feel hunger and perhaps this is why she regularly drinks amniotic fluid from which she derives both water and some nutrition. It is one of the ways in which the fluid gets used up, while it is continually replenished and freshened. This is not a stagnant pool and about a third of its volume is exchanged every hour.

The baby needs to gain more than a pound in the sixth month, and close to two pounds per month thereafter, to build up a sturdy birth weight. How tall she will be at birth is controlled almost entirely by her genetic program, but how much weight she now gains depends greatly on the efficiency of the placenta and on the mother's available stores. The latter rely not only on what the mother is eating now but also on how well nourished the mother has been all through her life. This is why long-term poverty and deprivation tend to be associated with "small-for-dates" babies who usually tend to be much more vulnerable.

In gaining weight, the baby becomes more rounded as she begins to put on an important padding of fat. Some of the fat will be a special kind named "brown fat" because it has a brownish color. Hibernating animals have this special fat, people have it around the newborn period. In addition to providing insulation, brown fat itself produces heat. Like built-in heating pads, this fat will help to keep the baby warm in the early weeks after birth. The special brown fat develops in just three areas: at the nape of the neck, around the kidneys, and behind the breastbone. At the same time, layers of ordinary white fat also appear and will give a cushioning and insulating padding, helped by the skin, which now turns into a thicker covering. But skin pigment is not yet distributed, so that dark- and light-skinned babies look alike at this age.

The baby starts to look slightly plump and becomes increasingly solid. The skeleton continues to harden, incorporating calcium, as do the toenails and fingernails which become harder and longer. Hair begins to grow out, first on the eyebrows and eyelashes, followed in the sixth month by head hair, to be short and wispy, or even quite full and long at birth.

A temporary provision of hair also develops. In the fifth month a fine, colorless fuzz appears all over the body. It is called *lanugo*, from the Latin word for wool. The woolly lanugo will last only for the next three or four months and will be mostly shed before birth. It has been suggested that lanugo might have a useful function, to trap and keep in place the coating of thick white cream that emerges on the skin at the same time. The cream is called *vernix,* meaning varnish, and it thoroughly covers the skin. It is an excellent, self-provided protection for the more finished skin against damage from the immersion in fluid in the coming months. Babies bring vernix with them at birth, especially in creases and folds where it has not rubbed off.

During the sixth month, the baby comes to the edge of being able to survive if born, but she would have only a frail grip on life and would need much intensive medical care. Such early birth is always a setback and these babies do not give us a true picture of the thriving unborn. Early-born babies do tell us that at this age the vocal cords can function; prematurely born babies can cry weakly, and show stress responses under conditions that might cause pain.

In the womb the baby must have the same capacities to feel discomforts but without air she of course cannot cry. Although life in the womb is not a perfect paradise, the baby profits enormously by staying there for the next three months. In that time she will become remarkably competent and well prepared for birth.

A fine fuzz soft lanugo on face and body will be mostly shed before birth. Lashes grow on eyelids, here still sealed.

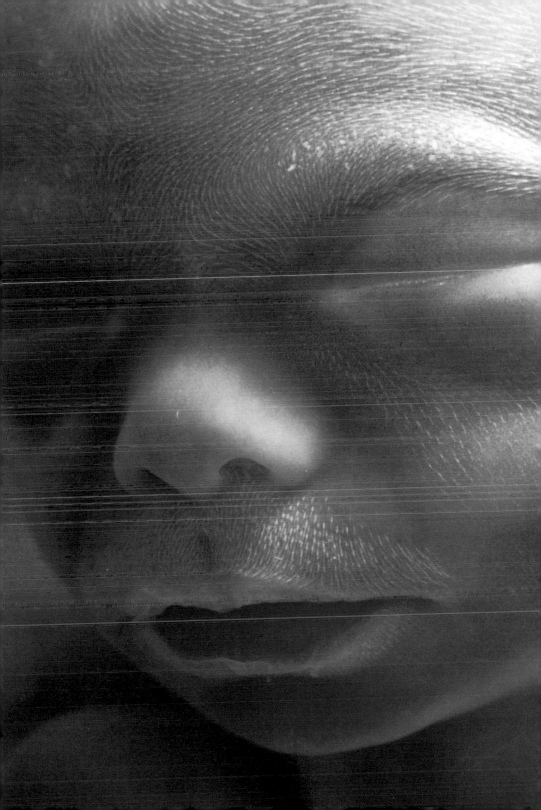

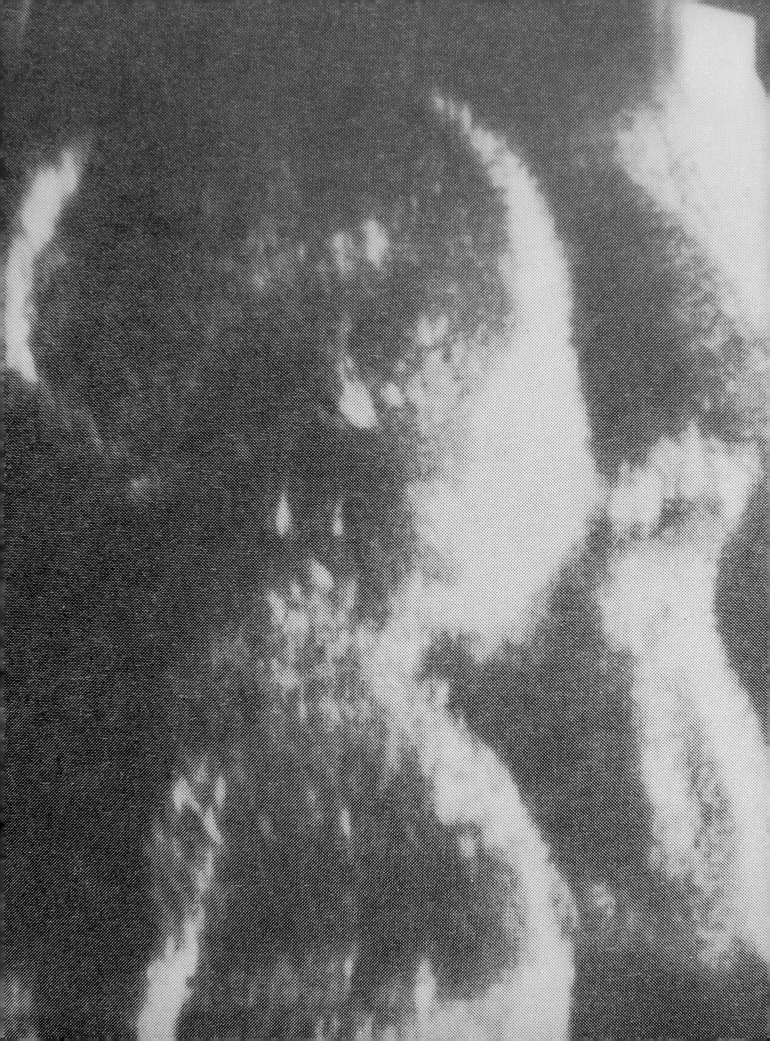

The baby outgrows her room in these three months and becomes ready to move out. Early in the seventh month there is still space enough for her to straighten up,

The seventh, eighth, and ninth months

Upright and skilfully putting hand to mouth at seven months, seen by ultrasound.

as she expertly puts her hand to her mouth, probably to suck her thumb. Her eyes are open, her eyelids are fringed with lashes, and she often moves her eyes as if searching for something to see.

She may as before experience an occasional faint orange glow if her mother is standing in any light bright enough to filter through the abdominal wall. It is possible that the baby may be able to see shadowy silhouettes of her surroundings in the womb. Certainly her senses become well developed and engaged in experiencing her environment. Her hearing is excellent and she becomes a listening member of her family. At birth she will probably be able to recognize her mother's voice, and favor it, but will give close attention to other people also. This attentiveness tends to help a baby attract the loving care she needs when born. Being appealing and lovable will be as important to the baby as her physical readiness for birth. She will need a lot of help.

In recent years we have come to recognize how much babies already know by the time they are born. Much of this is learned in the three months before birth, when the most studied of the baby's channels of learning is her hearing. The baby is continually surrounded by sound. There is the steady boom of the mother's heartbeat, the churning of the mother's digestion, the rushing of the bloodstream through the mother's large vessels, and the throbbing umbilical cord, always within earshot. All these produce a constant wash of sound. It may be similar in effect to the pounding ocean at the seashore to which one can become so accustomed that it fades into the background. It has been established that above the internal background noises the baby can hear people when they are talking in ordinary conversational tones. Voices come across through the mother's abdominal wall. Not word for word, but some words quite clearly, and altogether the rhythm and melody of speech. We know that she can also hear many of the prominent sounds of the immediate neighborhood. The baby reveals that she has heard by responding in ways that can be monitored. She may suddenly move more, her heart may suddenly beat faster, she may change her breathing, or she may blink her eyes at any sudden loud noise.

Foremost, the baby learns to know her mother's voice because she hears it more often than any other speech and also because women's voices are in a range most audible against the internal background noises. Every time the mother speaks, the voice is projected as powerfully down into the body as it is broadcast outward. What the baby receives is somewhat muffled and distorted but still about as recognizable as a voice on a poor telephone connection might be.

In the very first hours after birth, babies can give evidence that they know their own mother's voice, and like it better than any other. Newly born babies can collaborate in such studies because they are not only able to suck on a rubber nipple, they can also alter their sucking rhythm for a reward: in this case not food, but the reward of hearing a tape of their mother's recorded voice. The set-up offered babies a choice of two tapes, one with a friendly greeting recorded by their mother, the other carrying the same

Born early
at seven months, at her mother's breast, this baby shows how capable a baby can be at this age.

friendly words but recorded by another mother, addressing her own baby. By altering the sucking rhythm on the rubber nipple, babies could switch channels and choose to hear one tape or the other. It turned out that babies significantly preferred the taped voice of their own mother. This proved that they could distinguish one female voice from another, and they gave top rating to their own mother's speech.

Along with getting to know the mother's manner of speaking, the prenatal baby also picks up the characteristics of the local language. In studies carried out with French-speaking mothers it was found that right after birth their babies, apart from preferring their own mother's voice, preferred to listen to a French-language tape rather than a Russian one. These babies seemed to demonstrate that they had learned to distinguish the general sound of one language from another; apparently they had already developed an ear for their mother tongue. They had good preparation for the language they will want to understand and speak.

In the last months before birth, the baby may also learn to recognize passages of music or catchy texts repeatedly heard. The psychologists testing this used three children's stories: *The Cat in the Hat* and alternatively *The King, the Mice, and the Cheese,* as well as a story which the investigators themselves invented, called *The Dog in the Fog.* From the seventh month of pregnancy onward, a group of mothers each read aloud an assigned set of passages from only one of the books. Each pregnant mother recited the story in a normal speaking voice and did this regularly every day until birth. When born, their babies indicated recognition by becoming especially alert, or becoming quiet when crying, when they again heard the particular passages from the chosen book. But they did not pay this sort of attention to the sound of the equally catchy stories that had not been read to them before birth.

The baby may similarly learn to recognize music by hearing it before birth. For this investigation, pregnant mothers repeatedly played certain passages from the children's classic *Peter and the Wolf*. The bassoon sections were chosen because this instrument is in a range likely to be most clearly received by the baby. Indeed, when born, the babies appeared to show familiarity with this music and paid special attention to it. The same may also happen if a pregnant mother often hums a tune, or listens to it, so that the baby hears it over and over again. This has been investigated with the distinctive signature tune of an Australian TV series called *Neighbours*. A group of pregnant mothers regularly watched the program. When

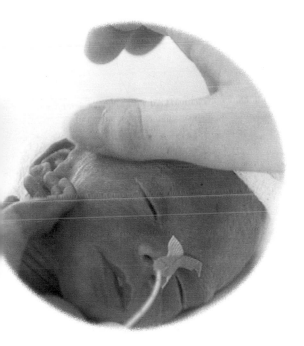

In an incubator
in the eighth month the baby is frail and less vigorous than she would be in the womb.

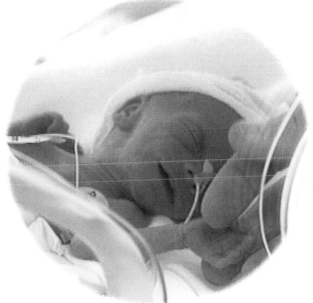

Smiling faintly
with a tiny hand laid in her mother's, she prospers under her mother's tenderness.

their babies were born, and then heard the signature tune, they became more alert, or stopped crying, and tended to show what has been jokingly described as "early soap addiction." It is thought possible that the pregnant mothers' comfortable state of relaxation while enjoying a favorite pastime might somehow have been transmitted to their babies. Therefore it might have been the feeling of relaxation, as well as the charm of the tune, that formed a pleasant association for their babies.

Kin recognition familiar from within with her mother's voice, her warmth, and perhaps even the taste to be found in her milk.

Before birth, when babies hear speaking voices, vowels are the sounds most clearly transmitted. So the "oohs" and "aahs" with which adults often greet newborns may be welcome because such sounds are already familiar to the baby. Altogether, prenatal learning appears to serve babies in "kin recognition." They learn to recognize their tribe. This can give them a good start toward feeling at home when born, toward fitting in with their particular family and local culture, and oriented toward making friends in that circle. The familiarity may extend even to the ingredients of home cooking. There is evidence that aromatic flavors, such as garlic or curry spices, may reach the baby in the womb, either via the umbilical cord or the amniotic fluid. There are indications that newborns may prefer their breast milk to be plain, or to contain hints of garlic, or spices, according to what the mother habitually ate during pregnancy.

Babies have more taste buds before birth than they will have later in life. They also appear to have a sweet tooth. This is known from an unusual medical treatment given to two mothers in the 1930s to reduce a troublesome excess of amniotic fluid. A sweetened solution was injected into the amniotic fluid, and this successfully enlisted the babies in drinking up the excess.

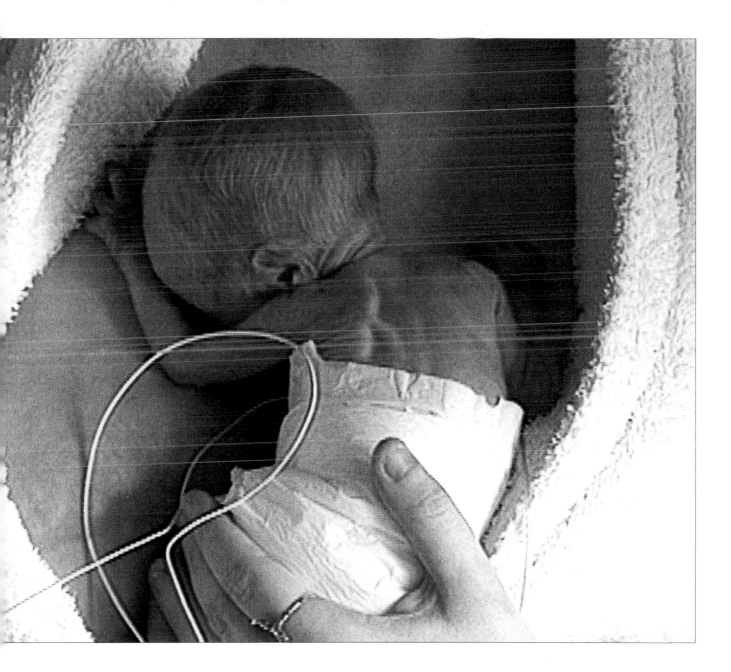

Normally, in the seventh month, the one-quart volume of amniotic fluid is reduced by half. How this happens remains to some extent a puzzle. It is a necessary adjustment since the growing baby needs the extra space, but at the same time she loses the former buoyant freedom. She can no longer move so extravagantly. For the mother, the reduction of cushioning fluid means that she can feel the movements more and anyone looking at her bare belly can see the undulations of the hidden baby's kicks and turns. If the mother takes a warm bath these activities may increase and make waves in the bathwater. Perhaps the baby is motivated by feeling some of the mother's ease in the bath; it is even considered possible that the warmth of the water may be transmitted. If the commotion makes the mother laugh, the baby gets jiggled, the movements increase, and the waves get going all the more.

The bouncy baby could live increasingly well if born prematurely. But until the last weeks, generally until she weighs about five pounds, she would still be frail in the struggle to survive. She would need the support of medical care. She might have difficulty with breathing; her lungs might not be ready to stay expanded to deal effectively with oxygen; she will probably require tube feeding, and she may at first lose weight when she most needs to gain it. She may need to be constantly warmed in an incubator. One of the pleasantest experiences for her would be

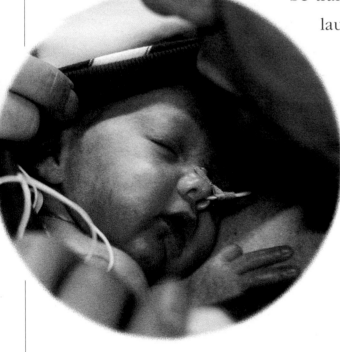

"Kangaroo care"
cozy inside the father's shirt, a premature baby receives the incubating warmth she still needs.

to be cuddled "kangaroo" fashion for the warmth she needs, which her father can provide equally well.

The baby who remains inside is much more vigorous. As the nervous system becomes more mature, the daily ups and downs of her activities tend to become more pronounced and regular. Relatively restful mornings may become more clearly distinguished from more active afternoons and evenings. The baby's measurable heart rate also begins to have clearer ups and downs according to her activities and experiences. With increasing maturity she develops a difference between sleep and waking. Yet being asleep does not mean lying still. The baby may toss and turn during a large part of her sleep while her eyes also move under closed lids. This is REM sleep, standing for rapid-eye-movement sleep, which all children and adults also have, usually accompanied by dreaming. Who knows, the baby too may dream of sounds, of tastes, of pleasures, or even fears?

Sleep and waking become more differentiated toward the end of the eighth month. Four distinct behavioral states become recognizable and these will continue to be characteristic in the baby's behavior in the weeks beyond birth. In sleep, the active state with rapid eye movements continues to predominate. In the briefer periods of quiet sleep, the baby does not move, not even her eyes. When the baby is awake, she opens her eyes and she may also be either active, or almost motionless and quiet. Being quietly awake is the most alert and attentive state, and is a baby's best time for learning. Being actively awake is the time for athletics, kicking and turning, insofar as this is still possible in her crowded quarters. At birth, only one more behavior will

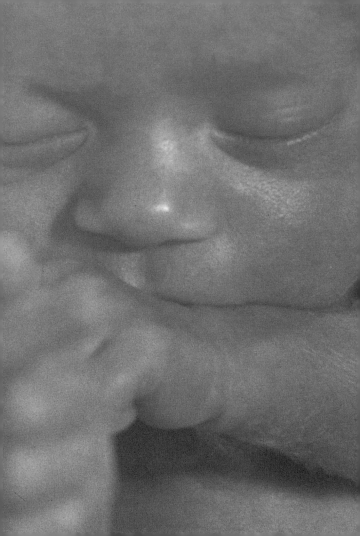

be added. This is crying, although that may not be the first time the baby could have cause to complain.

In becoming ready for birth the baby gains the bulk of her birth weight. For boys the average is near eight pounds, for girls it is seven. Most of this is put on in these final three months. Early in the seventh month the baby may weigh close to two pounds. She then quickly gains about two more pounds during the seventh month, and two more in the eighth. In the ninth month she is likely to add only one pound because she will get less nourishment from the aging placenta in the run-up to birth. An essential part of her weight gain, about one pound of it, is laid down as covering fat which will help to keep her warm. It will also make her more attractive to our eyes as her body becomes more chubby. Her face fills out more as her cheeks fatten up, adding to the fullness of her powerful sucking muscles. These efficient cheeks will be a prominent feature of her pleasing baby face.

Fat cheeks she gains her chubby baby face in the ninth month.

One of the best parting gifts the baby receives from her mother in the final months of pregnancy is an array of substances that combat diseases. These are large protein molecules called antibodies, taken up by the placenta from the mother's bloodstream and transferred to the baby. Some of the mother's antibodies may also enter the amniotic fluid and in this way reach the baby when she regularly drinks the fluid.

Antibodies are available for all of those diseases to which the mother has become immune in the course of her life. These may include measles, mumps, chicken pox, whooping cough, scarlet fever, influenza, the common cold, and numerous major and minor infections. If the mother has been effectively vaccinated against polio,

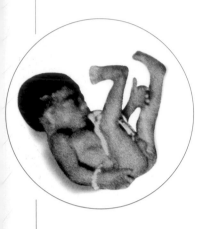

or smallpox, antibodies against those diseases are also passed on. The protection the baby gains will be good but not perfect and it will last for only about six months. This will tide the newborn over while the infant immune system gains competence. The mother's breast milk will also carry antibodies and these will boost the baby's resistance to infections when she drinks the milk.

The baby has a say in setting her own birth date. Although labor can be induced artificially, the normal process is different, and so complex that it still eludes complete understanding. It seems clear that in the normal process some biochemical, hormonal signals come from the baby when she has reached a certain level of maturity. These substances from the baby contribute to the running down of the functions of the placenta, leading to a chain of hormonal events. These become the trigger for the huge upheaval of labor. It is time to move out.

By this time, the baby has taken up her position for birth and probably got herself there by her own efforts, perhaps a month or perhaps only days in advance. For most babies, about ninety percent of them, this will be head-down which is the easiest way to get out. Ideally, her head is at the outlet, and her bottom and folded legs are accommodated in the wide arc of the top of the uterus. She can no longer move very much. She may achieve this position because she has reflexes to make small stepping movements and also to push off with her feet if her soles contact a firm surface. In the tight space of the womb her feet are very likely to encounter the firm wall of the uterus, setting off her stepping movements

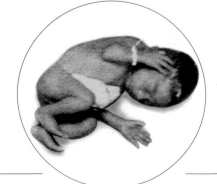

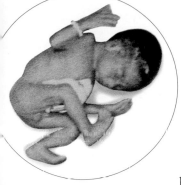

until one day, when she has become too big to maneuver, her head may get stuck in the dip that is the opening to the birth canal. This is the cervix. As her feet push, her head becomes well lodged in the exit and she cannot get out again. This is her "engagement" for birth. When her head becomes engaged in the cervix, her mother will probably feel the "lightening" as the mass of the baby sinks lower.

Acrobatics
a premature baby demonstrating what any baby may attempt in the restricted prenatal quarters, sometimes landing in an awkward position for birth.

Some babies get into different positions, sometimes quite awkward ones. They may get their buttocks engaged in the outlet for a breech birth; they may lie like a jackknife with their legs straightened; they may lie with back and head arched backward. For easier birth, it may be possible to coax them out of these less desirable positions by various traditional strategies of gentle external manipulation, or prescribed maternal positions, or rotation by more invasive medical intervention. But babies may insist and go back to where they were.

When the baby is in her starting position for birth she is at the very place where the sperm entered nine months ago to fertilize the egg. The spark of life has given way to hundreds of millions of cells. Together these weigh about two billion times more than the fertilized egg. Huge as these numbers are, they do not begin to describe the enormity of the transformation from one cell into the small person about to be born.

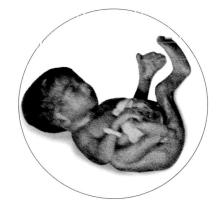

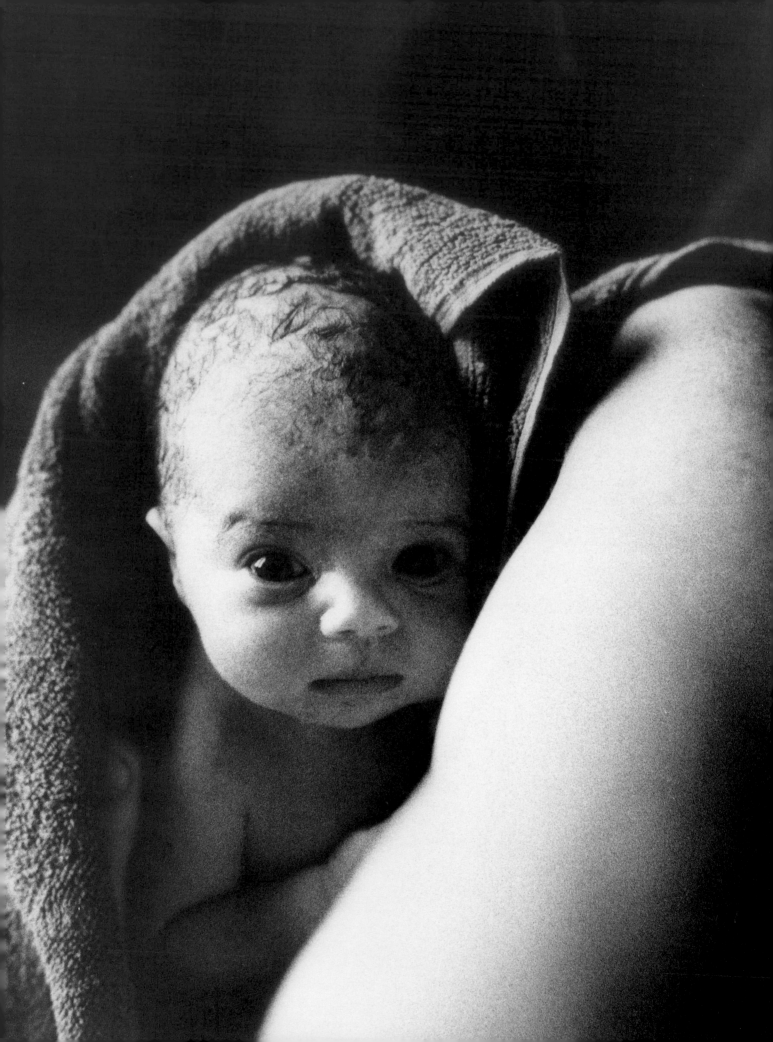

Birth can be an exciting experience for the baby. It is arduous, yet so stimulating that this little girl is radiantly wide awake a few minutes after being born.

The day of birth

... no more their wonted joys afford the fringed placenta and the knotted cord.

Oliver Wendell Holmes

She is still wet as she is received into the arms of her mother and with wide-open eyes takes in the one whose voice she already knows so well.

Just born and wide awake.

One may imagine the new sensations flooding the baby: the bright surprise of light, the new sights, the familiar sounds and new sounds, the chilly air after the near one-hundred-degree climate she has just left, air coming into her nose, the heaviness of gravity, the sudden clumsiness of her own body, the open space. And there are also the major changes within her own body as her lungs become inflated and her circulation is rerouted to take over from the umbilical cord. Her heart may beat quite fast and she is altogether aroused by the effects of birth. In the shower of new impressions she will probably stay awake and especially alert for most of her first hour out in the world.

The time for being born usually begins at night. The mother's body responds to the hours of darkness and there appears to be a physiological response that favors night as the time for the muscles of the uterus to start the labor of pushing the baby out. Sometimes there are false starts, mere rehearsals, giving both mother and baby an inkling of what is to come.

When real labor begins it keeps going and will have two distinctly different stages. In the first and longest stage, the baby stays put. This is the stage when the narrow entrance to the uterus, the cervix that admitted the microscopically small sperm, becomes opened to let the baby out. For the great majority this progresses slowly and smoothly over many hours. In the process the baby is like a wedge, stretching the exit to the size required. The power behind the baby is supplied by the formidable muscles around the top of the uterus. These create a downward thrust, which gradually builds up to be comparable to a weight of fifty-five pounds applied to the baby with each contraction. The baby may help somewhat by continuing to push off against the top of the uterus. The mother can help primarily by being relaxed, not flat on her back, but walking or otherwise moving around in ways that allow the process to have the pull of gravity on its side. If for any reason the exit cannot become large enough, the only alternative route out would be by cesarean surgery, which is a lot faster but not easier on the baby than ordinary labor. Babies are fitter and livelier after the more gradual process of uncomplicated birth, and the massage of labor may have a good effect.

In the process of normal birth, the baby's head can best take the leading part. The head has the largest diameter of the body and therefore once it is through, the rest can follow. Also, the head is well adapted to forge the way. The skull is made of five bone plates that are not yet fused together. The spaces between the skull plates are the fontanels, or "little fountains," which are the pulsating soft spots that can be felt on the head of any young infant. The fontanel gaps allow the skull plates to become pushed together, sometimes even to overlap, and this can reduce the circumference of the head by as much as an inch in the course of birth. In this way the round head can become temporarily and safely molded into a more elongated shape to suit the birth canal. When the head passes through the cervix, this might be compared to getting through a very tight turtleneck that cannot stretch beyond the size

Molded head
the newborn's elongated head is a reminder of its passage through the birth canal. The head will gradually round out again

of the surrounding bone circle of the mother's pelvis. When this obstacle is passed, the baby can begin to leave the uterus. This is the transition to the second stage of labor.

In leaving the womb, the baby drags her umbilical cord along. The cord continues to be her lifeline to the placenta, which remains anchored in the uterus for the time being. But the baby, with rare exceptions, is no longer enclosed in the amnion, and is for the first time lying bare and close against her mother's tissues. Usually, the "water breaks" in labor and the baby is then awash in what may be a gush or only a trickle of fluid. This may help to smooth the way, along with the convenient slipperiness of the baby's vernix cream. The progress is a shared enterprise for mother and child. If it is unduly difficult for one, the other has some experience of that too. If the mother is receiving anesthetics, an equal dose is delivered to the baby through the cord and both of them will be affected by it.

In the second stage of labor, the baby must tunnel through the birth canal and travel a distance of about four inches. It is a tight squeeze all the way. This stage of labor requires a bigger push to move the baby, as the elastic tissues of the mother's vagina are stretched. The mother's whole body enters into a natural bearing down that supplements the power of the uterus to inch the baby along. If this does not work well enough, the more aggressive pull of forceps or a vacuum pump must be brought to the rescue.

The journey through the birth canal may take one to two hours but can safely take longer, or can sometimes be accomplished in record times of only ten or twenty minutes. Fast or slow, the baby is not merely a cumbersome bundle with a heartbeat. She may squirm; she may wriggle; she probably continues to push off with her feet;

she has reflexes that all go in the direction
of being moved along. She keeps up the occasional
practice of breathing movements that will stand her
in good stead when she eventually meets air.
Finally she gets there. Her head emerges. This is
called her "crowning" and it is indeed a glorious
moment of safe arrival, although her eyes are
closed, her face is squashed and fluid drips from her
nose. Then she may start to whimper gently or she
may silently and slowly draw her first breaths of air and
open her eyes, even before the rest of her body is born and
before she shows that she is a girl.

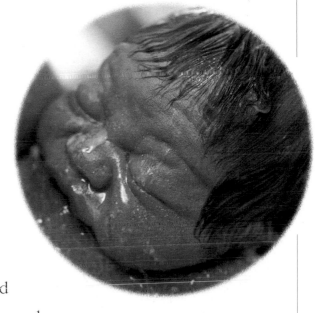

*The crowning
emerging like a
channel swimmer,
her face looks
squashed and
fluid drips from
her nose.*

    Her birth cry is brief, soft and pleasant, and usually brings smiles
to those who hear it. If the baby is gently received she is peaceful,
and perhaps she feels relief to be out. If she is chilly, she cannot
show it because she does not yet have the ability to shiver. She
depends on being offered extra warmth. If she cries lustily, she
is in discomfort but she has no tears as yet. The mild birth cry
is unlike any other crying and so individual for every baby that
recordings made of it are "cry prints" as distinctive as finger- or
footprints. Then, having made the modestly voiced announcement
of her arrival, the baby will start to look around – if she is at ease
and under comfortably low lighting.

    When she casts her eyes around they may move in unison but
occasionally lack coordination and veer off in opposite directions, to
briefly make her look cross-eyed or wall-eyed. The system needs
more tuning. She can see and can focus best on anything within
about half an adult arm's length from her. This suits her needs since

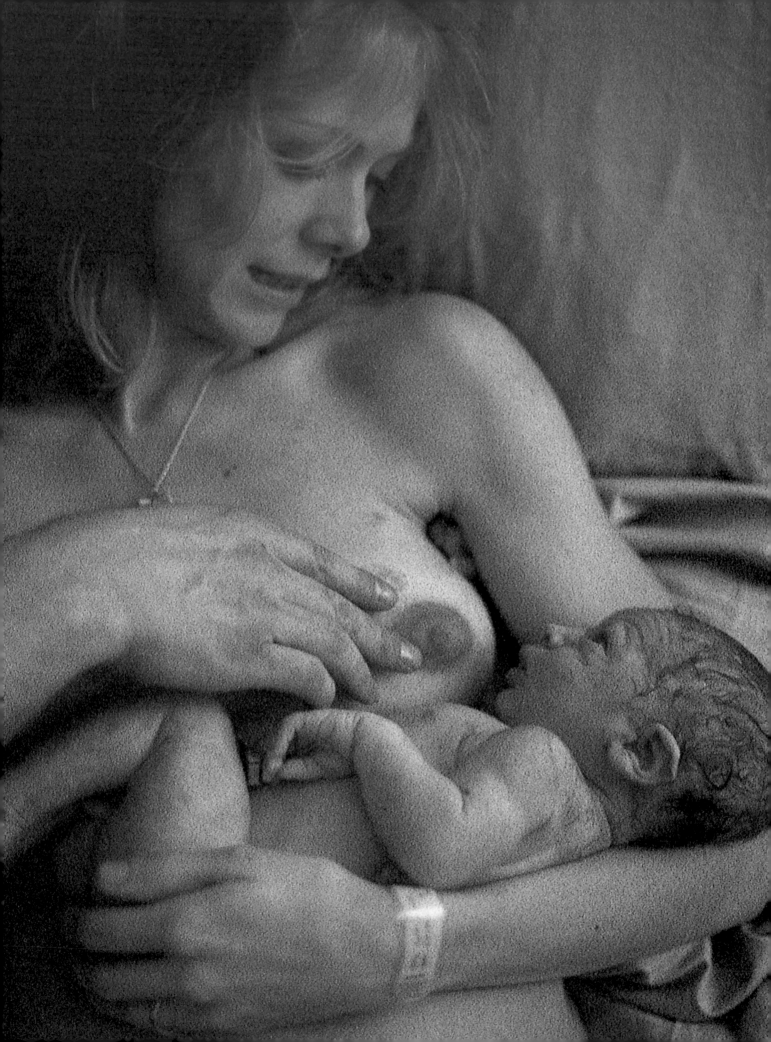

that is the very distance at which she often finds the thing of greatest interest to her: a human face. It is in her genetic makeup to be greatly attracted by faces. Any face, even a drawing of a face, may catch her eye and hold her attention. If the face moves to one side she will probably turn her head to keep watching. She likes to follow movement with her eyes while she cannot yet do it with her legs. She likes voices and if a voice calls she can detect the direction and usually tries to turn to it, slowly and hesitantly. She needs time and patience. Her responses may be fleeting and often so subtle that they appear vague. These are not yet the full-blown responses that will come later. If she is pleased she smiles, a modest and uncertain smile that is easily missed. She is a sociable being, she is attracted to people, and she needs people.

The ideal position to watch her mother's face, to listen to her voice, or choose to drink.

If the baby receives a warm response, her own responses bloom. The people in whom she is most likely to arouse the warmest feelings are her parents, so that a dialogue can begin wherein each arouses the feelings of the other. Fathers, mothers, and others become willing caretakers for such rewards. Nature does not rely on books to tell parents to care for their baby; the baby herself elicits our desires to watch over her and to take care of her. She benefits by being fed, held, carried, and kept warm. More than that, she also greatly profits because she is learning from people by paying such close attention to them. Being so helpless physically may have advantages for her social development because it brings her into close contact with people.

When her parents look at her, they will probably find her baby face pleasingly round. Her cheeks are full because she has such well-developed sucking muscles and needs them. She may have scratch marks on her face if her fingernails are long, as they often are, and the scratches are signs of her prenatal habit of touching and stroking her own face. She has a strong grip and the endearing ability to hang on tightly if offered a finger to hold. She has a reflex to close her hand if her palm is touched. Her hands are beautiful to watch. So small and yet so well formed and so "grown-up" and graceful in their activities as the fingers fan out and bend, open and close, reach and touch.

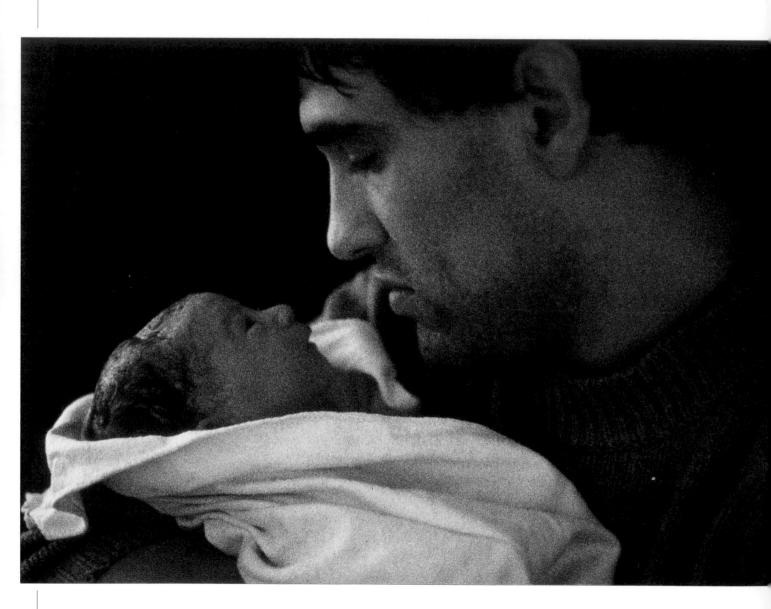

The father's rapt attention is returned by his child, just born. She can fully open her eyes only under dim light.

"It works!" is the frequent comment, very soon after birth, when the baby first urinates; it is an event somewhat more dramatic in boys than girls. Both a boy's scrotum and a girl's vulva are surprisingly large at birth. This is due to the effect of the hormones of pregnancy that the baby has shared. It is a temporary condition. The baby's breasts are similarly affected. The hormones that stimulated the mother's milk production reached the baby and also stimulated the

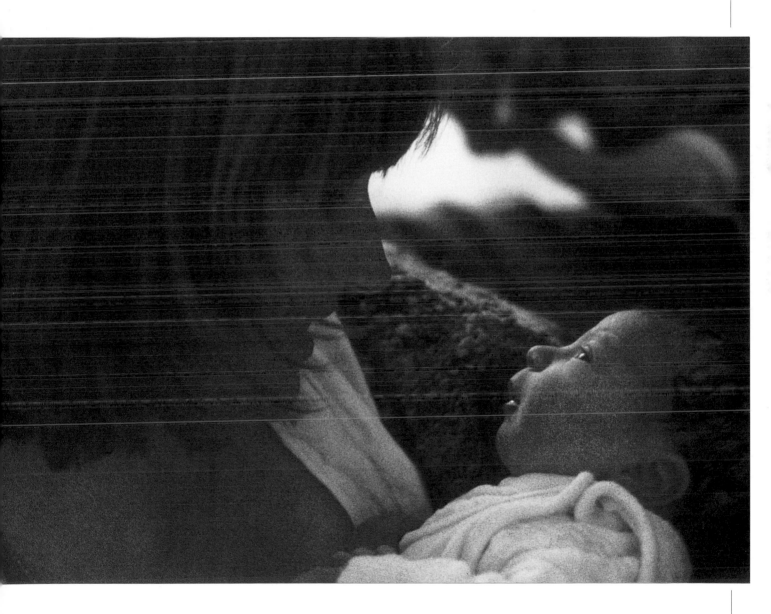

The mother's greetings are echoed by her baby's expression, and so a dialogue of sociable responses can begin.

baby's breasts. Therefore both boys and girls have drops of milk in their breasts for a few days after birth. Called "witches' milk," it may sometimes even leak from the nipples of the newborn. Thus even boys produce milk at one time in their lives.

These are short-lived links to prenatal life. So are remnants of creamy vernix and perhaps also some lanugo fuzz still on the back, shoulders, and forehead. From the long submersion, and the hours in birth, the baby's nose and throat and ears may be clogged with fluid and mucus. She coughs and sneezes and snuffles. She may occasionally pause in breathing and then breathe rapidly to make up for it. She did not need to breathe to get oxygen before.

The supplies through the umbilical cord stop very soon after the cord is exposed to air. A jelly-like substance within the cord swells up and shuts off the cord circulation. If the cord were not cut it would dry up and drop off in a few days. The baby needs the freedom to be picked up in arms, to suckle at the breast, to be face to face for this new phase of life.

She has arrived with vernix cream on the face, with good skills to try the breast, and the talent to engage her parents' caring attention.

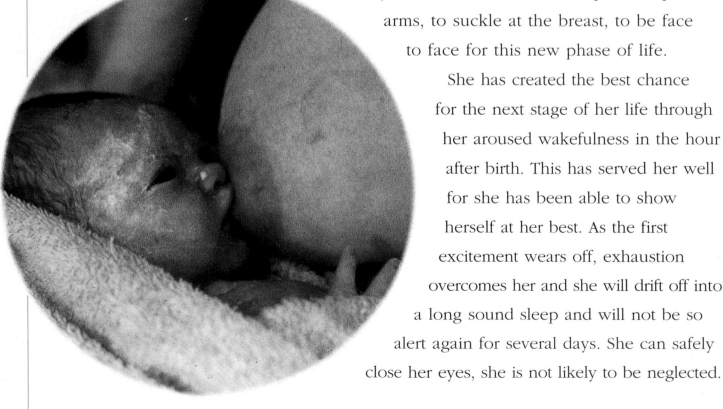

She has created the best chance for the next stage of her life through her aroused wakefulness in the hour after birth. This has served her well for she has been able to show herself at her best. As the first excitement wears off, exhaustion overcomes her and she will drift off into a long sound sleep and will not be so alert again for several days. She can safely close her eyes, she is not likely to be neglected.

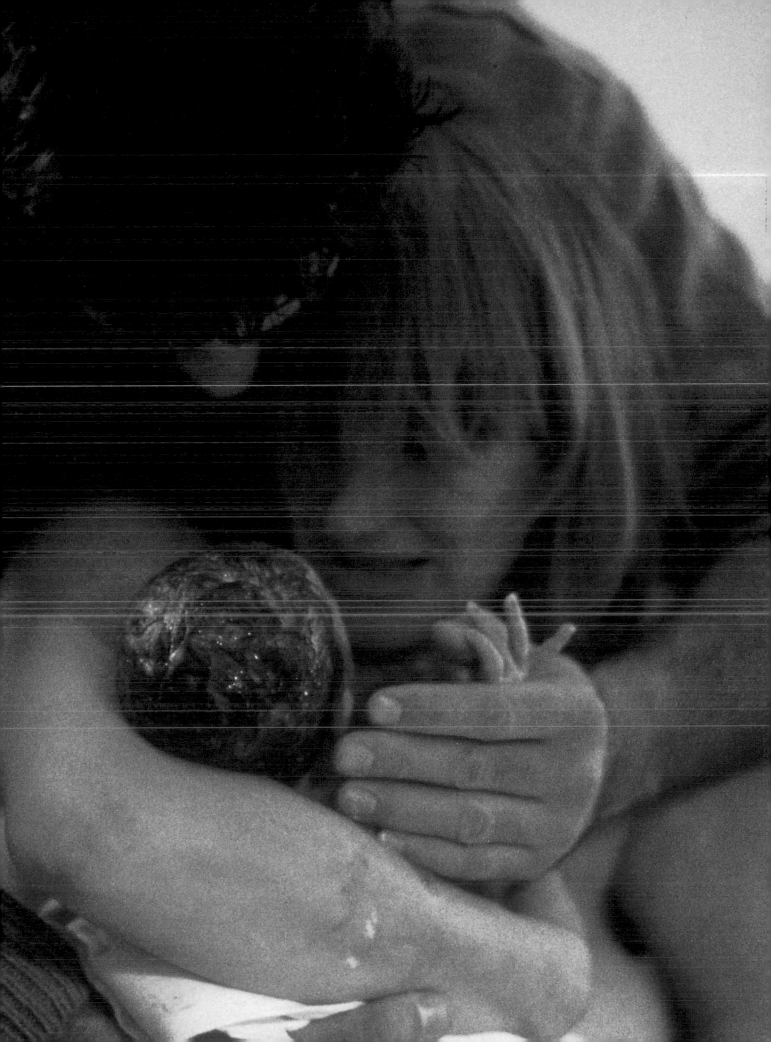

References for the text

GENERAL

ENGLAND MA 1990: A Colour Atlas of Life Before Birth: normal fetal development. *Wolfe Medical Publns, London.*

GILBERT SF 1991: Developmental Biology, *3rd edn, Sinauer, Sunderland MA, pp 66-154.*

MOORE KL, PERSAUD TVN 1993: The Developing Human: clinically oriented embryology, *5th edn, WB Saunders, Philadelphia, pp 29-112.*

FIRST DAY

Sperm

ABRAMOVICZ JS, ARCHER DF 1990: Uterine endometrial peristalsis - a transvaginal ultrasound study. *Fertility & Sterility 54:451-54.*

AITKEN RJ: Personal communication.

AITKEN RJ 1990: Evaluation of human sperm function. *Brit Med Bulltn 46:654-74.*

AITKEN RJ 1988: Assessment of sperm function for IVF *Human Reprodn 3:89-95.*

BAKER RR & BELLIS MA 1988: 'Kamikaze' sperm in mammals? *Animal Behaviour 36:936-39.*

BROMHALL D: Personal communication.

BROWN RL 1944: Rate of transport of spermia in the human uterus and tubes. *Am J Obstet & Gynecol 47:407-11.*

MORALES P *et al* 1988: Changes in human sperm motion during capacitation in vitro. *J Reprodn & Fertility 83:119-28.*

SETTLAGE DSF *et al* 1973: Sperm transport from the external cervical os to the fallopian tubes in women: a time and quantitation study. *Fertility & Sterility 24:655-61.*

Ovum

AITKEN J 1991: Do sperm find eggs attractive? *Nature 351:19-20.*

HÄGGSTRÖM P 1921: Zahlenmässige Analyse der Ovarien eines 22-jährigen gesunden Weibes. *Cited in Greenhill JP 1960: Obstetrics, 12th edn, WB Saunders, Philadelphia, p 5.*

MAKABE S, MOTTA PM 1982: Fetal Ovary. *In: Hafez ESE, Kennemans P (eds) Atlas of Human Reproduction by Scanning Electron Microscopy, MTP Press, Boston, pp 129-34.*

RALT D *et al* 1991: Sperm attraction to a follicular factor(s) correlates with human egg fertilizability. *Proc Natl Acad Sci USA 88:2840-44.*

SUNDSTRÖM P 1982: Interaction between spermatozoa and ovum in vitro. *In: Hafez ESE, Kennemans P (eds), Atlas of Human Reproduction, pp 225-30.*

Fertilization

DALE B 1991:Mechanisms of fertilization: plants to humans. *In: Neuhoff V, Friend J (eds), Cell to Cell Signals in Plants and Animals, NATO ASI Series, vol H51, Springer, Berlin, pp 83-90.*

EPEL D 1977: The program of fertilization. *Sci Am, Nov:128-38.*

ROBERTSON L *et al* 1988: Temporal changes in motility parameters related to acrosomal status: identification and characterization of populations of hyperactivated human sperm. *Biol of Reprodn 39:797-805.*

STOCK CE, FRASER LR 1987: The acrosome reaction in human sperm from men of proven fertility. *Human Reprodn 2:109-19.*

WASSARMAN PM 1988: Fertilization in mammals. *Sci Am, Dec:52-58.*

PLACHOT M, MANDELBAUM J 1990: Oocyte maturation, fertilization and embryonic growth in vitro. *Brit Med Bulltn 46:675-94.*

Cervical mucus

CHRÉTIEN FC 1982: Sperm cell-cervical mucus interaction. *In: Hafez ESE, Kennemans P (eds), Atlas of Human Reproduction, MTP Press, Boston, pp 219-22.*

DAUNTER B, LUTJEN P 1982: Cervical mucus. *In: Hafez ESE, Kennemans P (eds), Atlas of*

Human Reproduction, pp 55-59.

YUDIN AI *et al* 1989: Human cervical mucus and its interaction with sperm: a fine-structural view. *Biol of Reprodn 40:661-71.*

FIRST WEEK

Morula and Blastocyst

HARTSHORNE GM, EDWARDS RG [in press]: Early embryo development. *In: Adashi EY et al (eds), Reproductive Endocrinology, Surgery and Technology, Raven Press, New York, pp 435-50.*

BRAUDE P *et al* 1988: Human gene expression first occurs between the four- and eight-cell stages of preimplantation development. *Nature 332:459-61.*

DALE B *et al* 1991: Intercellular communication in the early human embryo. *Molecular Reprodn & Devpmt 29:22-28.*

DOKRAS A 1992: Human trophectoderm biopsy and its application. *D Phil Thesis, Oxford Univ.*

FULTON AB 1993: Small Wonder. *The Sciences, May/Jun:21-25.*

GLOVER DM *et al* 1993: The Centrosome. *Sci Am, Jun:62-68.*

HANDYSIDE AH 1990: Preimplantation diagnosis by DNA amplification. *In: Chapman M et al (eds), The Embryo: normal and abnormal development and growth, Springer, London, p 81-90.*

PLACHOT M, MANDELBAUM J 1990: Oocyte maturation, fertilization and embryonic growth in vitro. *Brit Med Bulltn 46:675-94.*

SATHANANTHAN AH *et al* 1982: Ultrastructural evaluation of 8-16 cell human embryos cultured in vitro. *Micron 13:193-203.*

Maternal tissues

SUNDSTRÖM P, NILSSON BO 1982: Postovulatory endometrium. *In: Hafez ESE, Kennemans P (eds), Atlas of Human Reproduction, MTP Press, Boston, pp 61-69.*

SUNDSTRÖM P 1984: Electron microscopy of human oocytes, cleavage stage ova and pre-implantation endometrium within an in vitro fertilization programme. *Thesis, Univ Lund.*

Production of hCG

AHMED AG, KLOPPER A 1983: Diagnosis of early pregnancy by assay of placental proteins. *Brit J Obstet & Gynecol 90:604-11.*

DOKRAS A *et al* 1991:The human blastocyst: morphology and human chorionic gonadotrophin secretion in vitro. *Human Reprodn 6:1143-51.*

DOKRAS A *et al* 1991: Human trophectoderm biopsy and secretion of chorionic gonadotrophin. *Human Reprodn 6:1453-59.*

LOPATA A, HAY DL 1989: The potential of early human embryos to form blastocysts, hatch from their zona and secrete hCG in culture. *Human Reprodn, 4th suppl:87-94.*

MORTON H *et al* 1977: An early pregnancy factor detected in human serum by the rosette inhibition test. *Lancet i:394-97.*

Early loss

BRAMBATI A *et al* 1990: Ultrasound and biochemical assessment of first trimester pregnancy. *In: Chapman M et al (eds), The Embryo, Springer, London, pp181-94.*

HARDY K *et al* 1989: The human blastocyst: cell number, death and allocation during late preimplantation development in vitro. *Development 107:597-604.*

HERTZ-PICCIOTTO I 1988: Incidence of early loss of pregnancy. *New Engl J Med 19:1483-84.*

LITTLE AB 1988: There's many a slip 'twixt implantation and the crib. *New Engl J Med 319:241-42.*

Twins

GILBERT SF 1991: Twins. *In: Gilbert SF, Developmental Biology, 3rd edn, Sinauer, Sunderland MA, p 97.*

SLACK JMW 1991: From Egg to Embryo: regional specification in early development, *2nd edn, Camb Univ Press, p 189.*

Implantation

KAVATS S *et al* 1991: Expression and possible function of the HLA-G α chain in human cyto-trophoblasts. *In: Chaouat G, Mowbray J (eds), Cellular and Molecular Biology of the Maternal-Fetal Relationship, Colloque INSERM/John Libbey*

Eurotext, 212:21-29.

SARGENT IL: Personal communication.

SARGENT IL *et al* 1993: The placenta as a graft. *In: Redman CWG et al (eds), The Human Placenta, Blackwell Scientific, Oxford, pp 334-61.*

FIRST MONTH

Cell organization, migration, communities

BEARDSLEY T 1994: Big-time biology. *Sci Am, Nov:72-79.*

DAVIDSON EH 1990: How embryos work: a comparative view of diverse modes of cell fate specification. *Development 108:365-89.*

FLANAGAN JG: Personal communication.

JESSELL TM, MELTON DA 1992: Diffuse factors in vertebrate embryonic induction. *Cell 68:257-70.*

KRUMLAUF R 1994: Hox genes in vertebrate development. *Cell 78:191-201.*

MCGINNIS W, KUZIORA M 1994: The molecular architects of body design. *Sci Am, Feb:36-42.*

MELTON DA 1991: Pattern formation during animal development. *Science 252:234-41.*

RAFF MC 1992: Social controls on cell survival and cell death. *Nature 356:397-400.*

ROBERTIS EM DE *et al* 1990: Homeobox genes and the vertebrate body plan. *Sci Am, Jul:26-32.*

Diary of development

COPP AJ 1991: Embryonic development: the origin of neural tube defects. *In: Chapman M et al (eds), The Embryo, Springer, London, pp 165-80.*

MOORE KL, PERSAUD TVN 1993: The Developing Human: Clinically Oriented Embryology, *5th edn, WB Saunders, Philadelphia, pp 75-92.*

STREETER GL 1942, 1945: Developmental Horizons in Human Embryos. *Age groups XI-XIV, Contributions to Embryology, Carnegie Institution of Washington Publns.*

SECOND MONTH

Diary of development

(as above and the following)

BIRNHOLZ J 1992: Smaller parts scanning of the fetus. *Radiol Clins N Amer 30:977-91.*

COWAN WM 1979: The development of the brain. *Sci Am, Sep:112-33.*

REECE EA 1992: Embryoscopy: new develoments in prenatal medicine. *Current Opinion in Obstet & Gynecol 4:447-55.*

REECE EA *et al* 1992: Embryoscopy: a closer look at first-trimester diagnosis and treatment. *Am J Obstet & Gynecol 166:775-80.*

STREETER GL 1948, 1951 (prepared by Corner GW, Heuser CH): Developmental Horizons in Human Embryos. *Age groups XV-XXIII, Contributions to Embryology, Carnegie Institution of Washington Publns.*

Alcohol, Smoking, Drugs

FORBES R 1984: Alcohol-related birth defects. *Public Health, London 98:238-41.*

IDÄNPÄÄN-HEIKKILÄ J *et al* 1972: Elimination and metabolic effects of ethanol in mother, fetus, and newborn infant. *Am J Obstet & Gynecol 112:387-93.*

LITTLE RE 1977: Moderate alcohol use during pregnancy and decreased infant birth weight. *Am J Public Health 67:1154-56.*

MAURER D, MAURER C 1988: The World of the Newborn. *Viking, New York, pp 20-28, 246-48.*

Movement

NIJHUIS JG (ed) 1992: Fetal Behaviour: developmental and perinatal aspects. *Oxf Univ Press.*

VRIES JIP DE 1992: The first trimester. *In: Nijhuis JG (ed), Fetal Behaviour, Oxf Univ Press, pp 3-16.*

VRIES JIP DE 1992: 1987: Development of specific movement patterns in the human fetus. *Thesis, Univ Groningen.*

VRIES JIP DE *et al* 1986: Fetal behaviour in early pregnancy. *Eur J Obstet Gynecol & Reprod Biol 21:271-76.*

VRIES JIP DE 1985: The emergence of fetal

behaviour II – quantitative aspects. *Early Human Devpmt* 12:99-120

VRIES JIP DE 1982: The emergence of fetal behaviour I – qualitative aspects. *Early Human Devpmt* 7:301-22.

THIRD MONTH
Movement
(as above and the following)

HUMPHREY T 1964: Some correlations between the appearance of human fetal reflexes and the development of the nervous system. *Prog Brain Research* 4:93-135.

PRECHTL HFR 1986: Prenatal motor development. *In: Wade MG, Whiting HTA (eds), Motor Development in Children:aspects of coordination and control, Nijhoff, Dordrecht, pp 53-64.*

PRECHTL HFR 1992: Some remarks on the neonate. *In: Nijhuis JG (ed), Fetal Behaviour, Oxf Univ Press, pp 65-72.*

Hiccups
DUNN PM 1977: Fetal hiccups. *Lancet* ii:505.

FULLER GN 1990: Hiccups and human purpose. *Nature* 343:420.

GOLOMB B 1990. Hiccup for hiccups. *Nature* 345:774.

LEWIS PJ, TRUDINGER B 1977: Fetal hiccups. *Lancet* ii:355.

Response to sound
HEPPER P, WHITE R 1991: The development of fetal responsiveness to external auditory stimulation. *Brit Psychol Soc Abstracts, p 30.*

FOURTH MONTH
Placenta and umbilical cord
BEACONSFIELD P et al 1980: The Placenta. *Sci Am, Aug:80-89.*

REDMAN CWG et al (eds), 1993: The Human Placenta: a guide for clinicians and scientists. *Blackwell Scientific, Oxford.*

Activities and individual differences
VISSER GHA 1992: The second trimester. *In: Nijhuis JG (ed), Fetal Behaviour, Oxf Univ Press, pp 17-25.*

VRIES JIP DE et al 1988: The emergence of fetal behaviour III. Individual differences and consistencies. *Early Human Devpmt* 16:85-103.

FIFTH AND SIXTH MONTHS
Hearing
BIRNHOLZ JC, BENACERRAF BR 1983: The development of human fetal hearing. *Science* 222:516-18.

BUSNEL MC, GRANIER-DEFERRE C 1983: And what of fetal audition? *In: Oliverio A, Zappella MM (eds), The Behavior of Human Infants, Plenum, New York, pp 93-126.*

HEPPER PG 1992: Fetal psychology: an embryonic science. *In: Nijhuis JG (ed), Fetal Behaviour, Oxf Univ Press, pp 129-56.*

LILEY AW 1972: The foetus as a personality. *Aust NZ J Psychiatry* 6:99-105.

QUERLEU D et al 1989: Hearing by the human fetus? *Seminars in Perinatology* 13:409-20.

SHAW KJ, PAUL RH 1990: Fetal responses to external stimuli. *Obstet & Gynecol Clins North America* 17:235-48.

WALKER D et al 1971: Intrauterine noise: a component of the fetal environment. *Am J Obstet & Gynecol* 109:91-95.

Activities
MAURER D, MAURER C 1988: The World of the Newborn. *Basic Books, New York, pp 7-31.*

ROODENBURG PJ et al 1991: Classification and quantitative aspects of fetal movements during the second half of normal pregnancy. *Early Human Devpmt* 25:19-35.

VRIES JIP DE et al 1987: Diurnal and other variations in fetal movement and heart rate patterns at 20 to 22 weeks. *Early Human Devpmt* 15:333-48.

Twins boxing; Earthquake effects
IANNIRUBERTO A, TAJANI E 1981: Ultrasonographic study of fetal movements. *Seminars in Perinatology* 5:175-81.

Eye movements and blinking
BIRNHOLZ JC 1985: Ultrasonic fetal ophthalmology. *Early Human Devpmt* 12:199-209.

BIRNHOLZ JC 1981: The development of human fetal eye movement patterns. *Science* 213:679-81.

INOUE M et al 1986: Functional development of human eye movement in utero assessed quantitatively with real-time ultrasound. *Am J Obstet & Gynecol* 155:170-74.

Maternal stress
BENSON P et al 1987: Foetal heart rate and maternal emotional state. *Brit J Med Psychol* 60:151-54.

BERGH BRH VAN DEN 1992: Maternal emotions during pregnancy and fetal and neonatal behaviour. *In: Nijhuis JG (ed), Fetal Behaviour, Oxf Univ Press, pp 157-78.*

STOTT DH 1973:Follow-up study from birth of the effects of prenatal stresses. *Devpmtl Med Child Neurol* 15:770-87.

Pain
ANAND KJS, HICKEY PR 1988: Pain in the neonate and fetus. *New Engl J Med* 318:1399.

ANAND KJS, HICKEY PR 1987: Pain and its effects in the human neonate and fetus. *New Engl J Med* 317:1321-29.

LANGLAND JT, LANGLAND PI 1988: Pain in the neonate and fetus. *New Engl J Med* 318:1398.

LAWSON JR 1988: Pain in the neonate and fetus. *New Engl J Med* 318:1398.

RICHARDS T 1985: Can a fetus feel pain? *Brit Med J* 291:1220.

SCHECHTER NL et al 1988: Pain in the neonate and fetus. *New Engl J Med* 318:1398.

SEVENTH, EIGHTH, AND NINTH MONTHS
Ability to hear
BENZAQUEN S et al 1990: The intrauterine sound environment of the human fetus during labor. *Am J Obstet & Gynecol* 163:484-90.

DIVON MY et al 1985: Evoked fetal startle response: a possible intrauterine neurological examination. *Am J Obstet & Gynecol* 153:454-56.

GAGNON R 1992: Fetal behaviour in relation to stimulation. *In: Nijhuis JG (ed), Fetal Behaviour, Oxf Univ Press, pp 209-26.*

GAGNON R 1989: Stimulation of human fetuses with sound and vibration. *Seminars in Perinatology* 13:393-402.

Speech and mother's voice
DE CASPER AJ, SPENCE MJ 1986: Prenatal maternal speech influences newborns' perception of speech sounds. *Infant Behavior & Devpmt* 9:133-50.

DE CASPER AJ, PRESCOTT PA 1984: Human newborns' perception of male voices: preference, discrimination, and reinforcing value. *Devpmtl Psychobiol* 17:481-91.

DE CASPER AJ, FIFER WP 1980: Of human bonding: newborns prefer their mothers' voices. *Science* 208:1174-76.

FIFER WP, MOON C 1989: Psychobiology of newborn auditory preferences. *Seminars in Perinatology* 13:430-33.

SHAHIDULLAH S, HEPPER PG 1994: Frequency discrimination by the fetus. *Early Human Development* 36:13-26.

Music
DAMSTRA-WIJMENGA SMI 1988: Fetal "soap" addiction. *Lancet* ii:223.

FEIJOO J 1981: Le foetus, Pierre et le loup. *In: Herbinet E, Busnel M-C (eds), L'aube des sens, Stock, Paris, pp 193-206.*

HEPPER PG 1988: Fetal "soap" addiction. *Lancet* i:1347-48.

NAIDOO N 1988: Fetal "soap" addiction. *Lancet* ii:223.

SHETLER DJ 1989: The inquiry into prenatal musical experience: a report of the Eastman project 1980-1987. *Pre & Peri-Natal Psych* 3:171-89.

Learning and kin recognition
HEPPER PG 1991: An examination of fetal learning before and after birth. *Irish J Psych* 12:95-107

HEPPER PG 1988: Adaptive fetal learning: prenatal exposure to garlic affects postnatal preferences. *Animal Behaviour*

36:935-36.

PORTER RH 1991: Mutual mother-infant recognition in humans. *In: Hepper PG (ed), Kin Recognition, Camb Univ Press, pp 413-22.*

Activities
HEPPER PG et al 1990: Origins of fetal handedness. *Nature* 347:431.

ISAACSON G, BIRNHOLZ JC 1991: Human fetal upper respiratory tract function as revealed by ultrasonography. *Ann Otol Rhinol & Laryngol* 100: 743-47.

NIJHUIS JG 1992: The third trimester. *In: Nijhuis JG (ed), Fetal Behaviour, Oxf Univ Press, pp 26-40.*

NIJHUIS JG et al 1982: Are there behavioural states in the human fetus? *Early Human Devpmt* 6:177-95.

PATRICK J et al 1982: Patterns of gross fetal body movements over 24-hour observation intervals during the last 10 weeks of pregnancy. *Am J Obstet & Gynecol* 142:363-71.

PRECHTL HFR 1992: Some remarks on the neonate. *In: Nijhuis JG (ed), Fetal Behaviour, Oxf Univ Press, pp 65-72.*

SADOVSKY E, POLISHUK WZ 1977: Fetal movements in utero. *Obstet & Gynecol* 50:49-55.

WOERDEN EE VAN, GEIJN HP VAN 1992: Heart-rate patterns and fetal movements. *In: Nijhuis JG (ed), Fetal Behaviour, Oxf Univ Press, pp 41-56.*

Sleep, waking, behavioral states
MIRMIRAN M 1986: The importance of fetal/neonatal REM sleep. *Eur J Obstet Gynecol & Reprod Biol* 21:283-91.

PATRICK J 1989: The physiological basis for fetal assessment. *Seminars in Perinatology* 13:403-08.

PILLAI M, JAMES D 1990: Are the behavioural states of the newborn comparable to those of the fetus? *Early Human Devpmt* 22:39-49.

PRECHTL HFR 1984: Continuity and change in early neural development. *Clinics in Devpmtl Med* 94:1-15.

Eye movements and visual capacity
FIELDER AR et al 1988: The immature visual system and premature birth. *Brit Med Bulltn* 44:1093-118.

HORIMOTO N et al 1990: Fetal eye movement assessed with real-time ultrasonography: are there rapid and slow eye movements? *Am J Obstet & Gynecol* 163:1480-84.

Taste and touch
DESNOO K 1937: Das trinkende Kind im Uterus. *Cited in Windle WF 1940: Physiology of the Fetus, WB Saunders, Philadelphia, p 100.*

HOOKER D 1952: The Prenatal Origin of Behavior. *Univ Kansas Press.*

DAY OF BIRTH
Onset of labor
KOOY B VAN DER 1994: Calculating expected date of delivery – its accuracy and relevance. *New Generation Digest, Natnl Childbirth Trust, Sep:2-5.*

SWAAB DF et al 1992: Development of the central nervous system. *In: Nijhuis JG (ed), Fetal Behaviour, Oxf Univ Press, pp 75-99*

Labor and birth
ENKIN M et al (eds), 1989: A Guide to Effective Care in Pregnancy and Childbirth. *Oxf Univ Press, pp 225-33.*

LAGERCRANTZ H, SLOTKIN TA 1986: The "stress" of being born. *Sci Am, Apr:92-102.*

The newborn
EMDE RN et al 1975: Human wakefulness and biological rhythms after birth. *Arch Gen Psychiatry* 32:780-83.

JOHNSON MH, MORTON J 1991: Biology and Cognitive Development: the case of face recognition. *Blackwell, Oxford.*

KLAUS MH, KLAUS PH 1985: The Amazing Newborn. *Addison-Wesley, Reading, MA.*

WASZ-HÖCKERT O et al 1968: The Infant Cry: a spectrographic and auditory analysis. *Clins in Devpmtl Medicine No. 29, Spastics Internatl Med Publns.*

Index

Acknowledgments

The help and encouragement I have received have been given with such personal generosity and warmth as to make my work a pleasure. I have benefited from many instructive and stimulating discussions with scientists and others. I have had invaluable advice and suggestions and thoughtful, often corrective, comments on my manuscript. I have deeply appreciated the photographs entrusted to me (detailed in the picture credits). To all – over two continents and eight countries – I am more grateful than I can begin to express here.

I am most conscious of my debt to the following: to Professor Jonathan Aitken for his vivid accounts of his research and the critical reading of relevant sections of my manuscript; to Dr Mark Cullen for allowing me to include his inspiring photographs, and Melinda Creel for her help so cheerfully given; to Dr Brian Dale for his unfailing helpfulness, his critical reading of sections of the manuscript, and his beautiful photographs; to Dr John Flanagan, for so carefully and critically reading the whole of the manuscript, and Cara Flanagan, for her expert comments on sections of it; to Dr Christopher McCready who, as close friend and biologist, gave me the great benefits of his clear thought, his skills, and care; to Dr Ian Sargent for his help so freely given, and for critically reading the whole of the manuscript, and leading me to important pictures; to Dr Hanneke de Vries for her careful comments on sections concerned with movement, and for delightful pictures.

I am also particularly grateful to: Dr Derek Bromhall for his personal help; Dr François Chretien for trusting me with his sole prints (and refreshing my French-speaking); Professor Yves Dumez, together with Professor Oury, for their fascinating pictures; Dr Murray Enkin, for kindly reading the birth chapter; Dr Marjorie England for her personal help; Dr Robert Forman, and Ceinwen Gearon, for allowing me to witness the "in vitro" drama of the dividing cells and for a lovely photograph; Dr Geraldine Hartshorne for the pleasure of her beautiful photographs; Eddy Maher for taking a photomicrograph for this book; Dr Per Sundström for his warmly given help in searching out the best of his photographs; Saskia van Rees for giving so much time to fulfilling my requests, and both to her, and to Anthea Sieveking, for photographing birth with such consideration for the comfort of the baby.

I also thank Vreni Booth and Nuala Moroney for their careful comments on the manuscript, and Viv Quillin, Mary Angus, and Annelie Rookwood for their enthusiasm, advice and critique.

Finally, I feel fortunate to have been able to work so closely with the superb team at Dorling Kinderseley. I thank Christopher Davis for his personal interest, and Gwen Edmonds for being such a considerate and careful editor. Caroline Hunt for her patient editorial assistance, Ann Kay for reading the manuscript, and Sandra Raphael for her help with the index. Also, Chloë Alexander for her creative work on the jacket, and Tassy King, Nicola Powling and William Mason for design assistance. It was fascinating to work with Jon Tubmen at Touch Animation who meticulously prepared some of the pictures for publication. Working together with Peter Luff on the final design of the book has been a privilege, education, and pleasure. I have so much enjoyed his creative ideas and thank him for being so receptive to mine.

Picture Credits

Every effort has been made to trace the copyright holders. Dorling Kindersley apologises for unintentional omissions, however, and would be pleased in such cases to add an acknowledgment in future editions.

Prof RJ Aitken, MRC Reproductive Biology Unit, Edinburgh 19 *br* / **Am J Obstet Gynecol** 166:777 Mosby-Year Book, Inc 46 / **Dr JD Bromhall** 66 / **Prof Stuart Campbell** 90 / **Carnegie Institution of Washington** 35, 39 *bl,* 39 *br* / **Dr FC Chretien,** Université Pierre et Marie Curie, Paris 18 *bl,* 18 *br,* 19 *bl* / **Collections:** A Sieveking 110, 114 / **MT Cullen, M.D.,** Dept of Maternal and Fetal Medicine, Florida Hospital, Orlando 48, 49, 50-51, 53, 55, 56, 58, 61, 64, 65, 70, 72, 75, 78, 80-81, 82 / **Dr Brian Dale,** IVF italy srl., Naples 28, 29 *br,* 33 *cr* / **Prof Y Dumez & Prof JF Oury** 52, 57 / **Gruner + Jahr AG & Co, Hamburg:** Picture Press, Uwe Ahrens 109 / **Dr R Forman,** London Gynaecology and Fertility Centre 22 / **GL Flanagan** 44 / **Dr D Hooker & Dr T Humphrey** 102, 103 / **Dr GM Hartshorne** by permission Lippincott-Raven Press 23, 25 *tr,* 30, 31, 32 *cl,* 32 *br* / **Prof E Ludwig,** Anatomisches Institut der Universität Basel 36 / **Oxford Medical Genetics Laboratories** 42, 43 / **Oxford Scientific Films:** D Bromhall 17, 76, 79, 89 / **Dr IL Sargent,** Oxford IVF Unit, Nuffield Dept Obstet Gynaecol, University of Oxford 29 *tl* / **Science Photo Library:** Latin Stock, Oscar Burriel 8; Petit Format, Nestle 45, 69, 84, 85, 100 / **Anthea Sieveking** 104 / **Frank Spooner Pictures:** Gamma, Dr Per Sundström 15, 21, 24, 26, 27 / **Dr Per Sundström,** CURA kliniken, Malmö *front cover,* 12, 14, 16 / **University of California,** San Francisco 71 / **Saskia van Rees,** Stichting Lichaamstaal 93, 95, 96, 98, 107, 112, 113, 115 / **Dr JIP de Vries,** Academisch Ziekenhuis, Vrije Universiteit, Amsterdam 54, 62-63, 86 / **Wolfe Medical Publications,** © 1985 Marjorie A England 41. **Author Photograph:** Susie Barker.

The publishers would like to thank the following for permission to use quoted material: Aldous Huxley the "Fifth Philosopher's Song" from *Leda Poems* published by Chatto & Windus used by permission of the Reece Halsey Agency in the USA, and Mrs Laura Huxley and Chatto & Windus in the rest of the world. Anthony Thwaite "To My Unborn Child" published by permission of Curtis Brown Ltd. on behalf of Anthony Thwaite.

DATE DUE

3-11-08			
	WITHDRAWN		

UNIVERSITY PRODUCTS, INC. #859-5503